Monetizing *Obesity* Medicine

A Doctor's Framework for Patient Success at Scale

DR. ASHLEY WHITE, MD, MPH

J.ROSS PUBLISHING

ISBN: 978-1-60427-216-1
e-ISBN: 978-1-60427-871-2

Printed and bound in the U.S.A. Printed on acid-free paper.

10 9 8 7 6 5 4 3 2 1

Library of Congress Cataloging-in-Publication Data can be found in the WAV section of the publisher's website at www.jrosspub.com/wav.

Direct all inquiries to J. Ross Publishing, Inc., 151 N. Nob Hill Rd., Suite 476, Plantation, FL 33324. For EU safety/GPSR concerns, email: gpsr@mare-nostrum.co.uk or contact: Mare Nostrum Group B.V, Doelen 72, 4831 GR Breda, The Netherlands.

Phone: (954) 727-9333
Fax: (561) 892-0700
Web: www.jrosspub.com

To Sabrina and Malcolm

Your book includes a year of the author's newsletter.

Every copy of **Monetizing Obesity Medicine**—any retailer, any format—includes 12 months of *The Clinical Last Mile*, the author's newsletter on the business and practice of patient success: weekly essays on the clinical last mile and monthly working tools built on this book's KPIs and the Canopy framework.

Claim your subscription at: https://www.ashleywhitemd.com/claim

CONTENTS

INTRODUCTION

When I started prescribing GLP-1 medications for obesity in 2021, I did not yet understand that the prescription was the easy part. The GLP-1s work as advertised; they help people lose weight. They also work in other unexpected ways: improving heart, liver, gut, joint, and brain health. GLP-1s are among the most important pharmacological advances of the century. Evidence of their importance in treating the most burdensome chronic diseases in the industrialized world has been clear for several years. Chapter 1 lays out that evidence in detail.

But almost no one is staying on them. Nearly two-thirds of people who start a GLP-1 for weight loss will stop within 12 months.[1] In two years, only 15 percent will still be taking them. Patients who stop will regain most of what they lost within the year. With that, any benefit to their health will slowly erode.[2]

The market's strategy for GLP-1s at scale has been to awkwardly retrofit the management of a complex lifelong disease into e-commerce systems purpose-built for selling sweaters, groceries, and other commodities.

The health system's strategy has been to pretend that obesity is not a real disease, like diabetes or hypertension, and pass on responsibility for owning it like a hot potato—leaving patients stuck with trying to figure it out on their own.

WHY THIS BOOK? WHY ME?

I hold two parallel lenses in obesity medicine. I practice it, and I also design large-scale digital clinical obesity programs. The market shapes the medicine, and vice versa. I hold the door open between the two worlds, and I am bullish on the very real alignment of clinical and commercial success.

I am a Canadian physician. I have practiced independently since 2017 in both family and emergency medicine. I have been board-certified in obesity medicine since 2021. In 2023, I founded The Shift Clinic, a primary care practice designed for people with obesity and complex metabolic disease. Since 2024, I have designed and run clinical obesity programs for three major digital health platforms across Canada. Holding both perspectives at once is what makes this book possible.

I began my career as a Senior Policy Analyst with the Public Health Agency of Canada and then ran health programs for the Aga Khan Foundation in Afghanistan. I completed my master's degree in public health before attending medical school. At its finest, public health is simplicity at scale: handwashing, seat belts, helmets, and mosquito nets. Quality public health interventions do not abandon principles of human behavior and basic hygiene to chase flashy technologies. Public health experts understand that technologies only work if humans actually want to use them and have a system in which to do so.

MY BOOK TITLE

The title of my book is intentionally provocative. Doctors are not supposed to talk about money. We are trained to stay close to the mission and leave markets to others. But I am standing inside a broken system with no way to deliver care except through imperfect markets. I cannot solve that here. What I can say is that doctors have to show up. Our ethics have to shape how this market gets built. We cannot keep hiding from it. In fact, I think we should be building it ourselves.

I gave the book this title because doctors see what other people cannot see from the seat we occupy. It is a trusted seat, and protecting it now means participating in conversations about money and markets rather than letting them happen without us, and without our patients.

THE ALIGNMENT

Quality obesity medicine, including GLP-1s, is the largest opportunity we will see in our careers to simultaneously improve population health and lower healthcare costs—but only if we build something new. The interventions that keep patients engaged in therapy and producing durable clinical improvement are also the ones that generate sustained revenue per patient and a profitable lifetime value. Patient success and customer lifetime value are the same thing, measured differently. This alignment is rare in medicine. This is also why the market has attracted as much capital as it has, with GLP-1s making headlines every single day as I write this book.

GLP-1s are projected to be a $100 billion category by the end of the decade.[3] Yet, Chapter 2 shows that only 3.4% of the total addressable market for obesity was captured by brand-name GLP-1s in 2025. Tens of millions of people in the United States would benefit from access to treatment right now and would need to continue that treatment in order for the forecasts to be realized.

THE VOID

The natural home for chronic disease management is primary care. But American primary care is in structural collapse. The absence of meaningful obesity medicine training in residency curricula makes guideline-directed obesity care effectively impossible during a primary care visit.

There aren't enough obesity medicine specialists to even make a dent in the demand. The American Board of Obesity Medicine has certified the field for just over a decade. Many of the certified specialists do not practice obesity medicine full time. It is a niche specialty for a pandemic-sized problem.

Into this void, digital health platforms have arrived. Some of what has been built is genuinely useful. The dominant business model, though, is extractive and shortsighted. This is where the alignment between markets and medicine can fray. But it needn't be inevitable in obesity medicine. In fact, reinforcing this alignment may be our only way through the void.

THE FRAMEWORK

This book is not a polemic anti-market tirade, although it contains material, namely math, that some companies will not enjoy reading. And I don't spare the health system—and certainly not its payers—from their part in the problem. The book is a framework, written for the people who want to build the next system with me. And for those who have the time horizons, capital, and accountability to actually do it.

Part I describes the U.S. market and the gap, and shows why the failure to capture the market is a systems failure, not a scientific one.

Part II turns to other industries, drawing lessons from Apple, Ticketmaster, Peloton, Fitbit, and Zara. These companies faced the question of how to retain customers in markets where retention is the only path to a sustainable business. They either solved it, partially solved it, or failed in instructive ways.

Part III is the solution architecture itself: The Canopy Framework. It is organized around seven components that form a configurable ecosystem for patient success at scale in obesity medicine.

Chapter 1 opens in my clinic with a new patient, Sarah. She has spent two decades trying to outwork her own biology, and she has lost. She wants to know if I can help. Yes, I can. This moment in medicine, which lets us make good on that promise for millions of patients across decades of care, is the subject of the rest of this book.

ENDNOTES

1. Rodriguez et al., "Discontinuation and Reinitiation of Dual-Labeled GLP-1 Receptor Agonists Among US Adults With Overweight or Obesity," *JAMA Network Open* 8, no. 1 (2025): e2457349, https://doi.org/10.1001/jamanetworkopen.2024.57349.
2. Wilding et al., "Weight Regain and Cardiometabolic Effects after Withdrawal of Semaglutide: The STEP 1 Trial Extension," *Diabetes, Obesity & Metabolism* 24, no. 8 (2022): 1553–64, https://doi.org/10.1111/dom.14725.
3. Goldman Sachs Research, "Why the Anti-Obesity Drug Market Could Grow to $100 Billion by 2030," Goldman Sachs Insights, October 30, 2023, https://www.goldmansachs.com/insights/articles/anti-obesity-drug-market.

DISCLAIMER

AUTHOR'S NOTE

The case narratives in this book are composites, fictionalized accounts, or based on real individuals, used with informed consent. In every case, names and identifying details have been substantially altered to protect privacy. No real person should be identifiable from the narratives presented. Where a scenario closely tracks a single individual, that person has consented to its inclusion in modified form.

DISCLOSURE OF CONFLICTS OF INTEREST

The author receives episodic honoraria for speaking engagements, time-limited consultancies, and participation on advisory panels from Novo Nordisk, Eli Lilly, Bausch Health, and Rhythm Pharmaceuticals. The author has no equity holdings, ownership interest, or other ongoing financial interest in any referenced pharmaceutical or digital health company, and has no other conflicts of interest to disclose. The opinions, analyses, and recommendations in this book are the author's own and do not represent the views of any of the previously mentioned companies.

MEDICAL DISCLAIMER

This book is written for product builders, policymakers, designers, healthcare professionals, executives, investors, and other readers interested in the business, delivery, and ethics of obesity medicine. It is not medical advice and is not a substitute for individualized clinical care. Readers seeking medical guidance for themselves or others should consult a qualified clinician. The author is a practicing physician in Canada. Nothing in this book establishes a physician-patient relationship between the author and the reader. The author accepts no responsibility for clinical decisions made based on the content of this book.

A NOTE ON AI TOOLS IN RESEARCH AND DRAFTING

The author used artificial intelligence (AI) tools as research and drafting aids in the preparation of this manuscript—particularly for source synthesis, draft generation, and editorial iteration. All ideas, frameworks, clinical reasoning, structural decisions, and authorial voice are the author's own. Drafts produced with AI assistance were substantially revised and mostly rewritten in the production of the final manuscript. The author takes full responsibility for the accuracy and substance of the content.

INDEX OF KEY PERFORMANCE INDICATORS

ACKNOWLEDGMENTS

Writing a book while raising small children, building a practice, and advising on digital health has not been done alone. Not even close.

First, my thanks go to my patients. None of you appear by name or story in these pages, and that was deliberate. But the trust you have given me over the years, the stories you have shared, and the patterns I have learned to see by sitting with you are the foundation of this work. I believe in your success, not narrowly in weight lost but in health gained on your own terms. This book is for you, and for the system of care you deserve.

To Sharon White, my mom: Thank you for showing up and stepping in so that I could finish this, for parenting my children and me at the same time, and for making it possible to cross this finish line.

To Wayne White, my dad: Thank you for letting me write about you. I hope the system can find its way to helping you the way I wish it would.

To Tyler White, my brother: Thank you for caring so much about our parents, for keeping an open mind about my work, and for always being the guy who does the right thing.

To Angela Woodcock, our Community and Growth Director, and cousin extraordinaire: You picked up an editor's hat that you had never worn before and made it fit. Without your willingness to step into an unfamiliar role and figure it out as you went, this project would not have crossed the finish line. Thank you for combing through text for days on end, and never once rolling your eyes about it.

To Chantelle Woodcock, Clinic and Business Director and beloved cousin: While I was deep in finishing this book, you made sure the ship kept moving. Thank you for keeping us afloat, for feeding me, for fighting for me, and seeing me with your *signature* rose-colored glasses.

To Jensen Pletch: Thank you for the countless hours you spent ensuring that every citation, every quote, and every reference in this book is accurate and sound. And for even more than that—for being an exceptional part of this team, for trusting what we are building, and for taking the road never traveled with me.

Thank you to Angela, Jensen, and Chantelle for caring as deeply about our patients as I do.

To Jane Depraitere: This book exists, in no small part, because of you. Your belief in me, in this team, and in the importance of this message never wavered. You gave days upon days of editing, guidance, and wisdom that I could not have afforded and would not have found anywhere else. You pushed me at exactly the moment I needed it most, and you understood—truly understood—why this book matters and what it is part of building. I find help very hard to receive, but yours made me feel confident and empowered.

To Krista Huszarik and Jessica Robinson: Thank you for reading the early chapters and giving me the momentum I needed when this book was still figuring out what it was. Please refuse to review chapters if I ever fathom writing another one before my kids are adults.

To the good Dr. Adam Abbs: Thank you for being a steady presence across the pond when I was not sure I was going to make it to the end of this. Thanks also for reading, listening, counseling, and for being a true confidant.

To Drs. Megha Poddar and Puneet Seth: Thank you for building something remarkable in nymble, for never taking your eyes off the patient success prize, and for letting this book be a place where you can be seen for the visionaries you are. Your product is quickly becoming my appetite stethoscope.

To Dr. Jeff Alfonsi and Elizabeth Choi: Thank you for letting me fangirl about RxFood on these pages, for taking my feedback eagerly, and for continuing to innovate. I cannot practice without RxFood now, so you will have to be enormously successful forever.

To Sara Kahn: Thank you for the hours and hours spent verifying sources for the first sample chapters in 2025, no questions asked. I hope you like where it ended up.

To Dr. Zal Phiroz: Thank you for showing such dignity and kindness when I decided to do this on my own.

To Stephen Buda and J. Ross Publishing: Thank you for taking a chance on a first-time author from Canada regarding a topic that refuses to recede from the headlines. Thank you for allowing me additional time to deliver something worth reading.

ABOUT THE AUTHOR

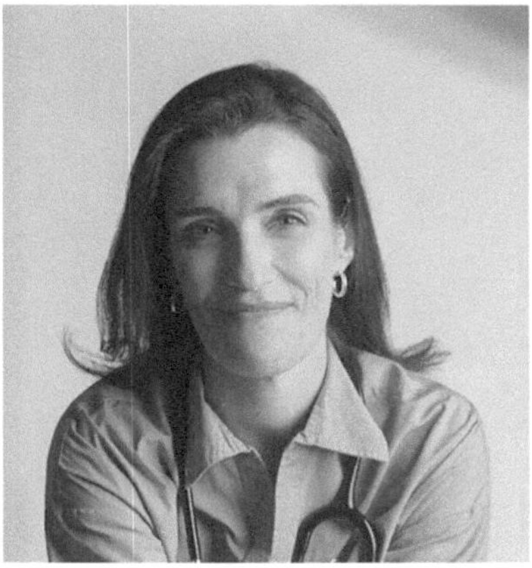

Dr. Ashley White is a Canadian physician with dual certifications: family and emergency medicine through the College of Family Physicians of Canada and a U.S. board certification in obesity medicine through the American Board of Obesity Medicine. She holds an MD from McMaster University, a Master of Public Health in global health from Simon Fraser University, and an Honours Bachelor of Arts and Science with a Minor in economics from McMaster. Her career began outside clinical medicine, first as a senior policy analyst at the Public Health Agency of Canada, then in health program implementation with the Aga Khan Foundation in Afghanistan, and later in inner-city health research. She has practiced family and emergency medicine in rural and urban Ontario since 2017. Since 2021, her clinical focus has been on obesity and metabolic health, which includes the patient population whose patterns inform every scene in this book.

She has been working from inside the digital health sector during the GLP-1 boom. In 2024 and 2025, she was Director of Women's Health and Obesity at PocketPills. She is currently the Medical Director for North America at HeliosX. The Shift Clinic is her active primary care practice for people with obesity and complex metabolic disease. The Shift Clinic is a living laboratory for innovation in ethical obesity care. The Shift is also where the Canopy was developed before becoming the framework that organizes this book. Ashley lives in Hamilton, Ontario, Canada with her family.

This book has free material available for download from the Web Added Value™ resource center at *www.jrosspub.com*

At J. Ross Publishing we are committed to providing today's professional with practical, hands-on tools that enhance the learning experience and give readers an opportunity to apply what they have learned. That is why we offer free ancillary materials available for download on this book and all participating Web Added Value™ publications. These online resources may include interactive versions of material that appears in the book or supplemental templates, worksheets, models, plans, case studies, proposals, spreadsheets and assessment tools, among other things. Whenever you see the WAV™ symbol in any of our publications, it means bonus materials accompany the book and are available from the Web Added Value Download Resource Center at www.jrosspub.com.

Downloads for *Monetizing Obesity Medicine* include a KPI Workbook and a Unit Economics Model, both ready to adapt with your own program data.

Part I

The Gap in Obesity Medicine

CHAPTER 1

MIRACLES AND MISCONCEPTIONS

"Tell me what to do, and I'll do it," Sarah says.

Sarah is a new patient referred to me for help with losing weight. She arrives with the data—*so much data*. On the desk between us:

- Spreadsheets of lab results, medical records, and calorie tracking data
- A list of meal-delivery services she's tried, each one annotated with start dates and reasons for discontinuation
- A training log from her sessions with her personal trainer, three times per week for the past 18 months, and body composition testing
- Notes on feeding and fasting strategies
- A large Ziploc bag with supplement bottles and medications
- Multiple feeds from her wearable devices, each scoring her body's function, all day and night

She walks me through the data and looks at me. "I've lost and regained the same 50 pounds over and over again. I can't keep doing it. None of the old things I used to do work anymore," she says, hinting at the real fear underneath all of it.

Sarah is 44 and a corporate vice president. Her phone is face up on the desk between us. It pings every few minutes with work notifications. She glances at it while I'm reviewing her chart, thumbs out a quick reply, and sets it down. Another ping. She picks it up again, types decisively, and puts it back. She's running her team from my exam room. I know that Sarah is trying hard enough. Sarah tries hard at everything. She is used to having all the answers or leading the charge to find them.

In my practice, I care for many people like Sarah. They've always got the data. And the same confusion about why so much effort has produced nothing sustainable. Always the same belief that there must be a secret waiting to be unlocked, some combination of macros or timing or supplements that will finally make the body cooperate. And always the fear: *What if I can't do this on my own? What if I'm broken? What if this is just always going to be how hard it is for me to stay healthy?*

It is far simpler to believe that the missing ingredient is discipline. Sarah knows what that is. She has lots of it. That's free and doesn't require a prescription for a drug that she must take forever. But her appetite is dysregulated, as is her metabolism. This is partially inherited. Her family history shows that every adult in her family has obesity. Over decades, her perception of hunger and fullness, of wanting and satiety, was further altered by diet and weight cycles, stressful experiences, periods of poor sleep, pregnancies, and unpredictable work travel. Without medication, her odds of reaching and keeping a normal body weight are less than 1 in 100.[1] Discipline is not the missing piece.

This disconnect between the biology of obesity and the story of personal failure shapes everything in this market. It determines how patients seek care, how insurers evaluate coverage, and how pharmaceutical companies position their products. It is why we have a health crisis affecting 42% of U.S. adults,[2] why obesity-related complications drive an estimated $173 billion in annual medical expenditures,[3] and why the pharmaceutical industry is sitting on a theoretically trillion-dollar asset[4] it can't figure out how to deliver.

To understand the market opportunity, we must first strip away the cultural baggage and look at the clinical reality. Obesity is a chronic, relapsing brain-and-body disease of energy balance.[5] It sits at the mouth of a raging river of chronic disease that includes diabetes, heart disease, sleep apnea, metabolic liver disease, and more.[6] When we treat obesity, we are not treating a number on a scale. We are treating the upstream cause of some of the most expensive conditions in modern healthcare.

WHY DIETS FAIL (IN BRIEF)

The human body fights hard in defense of its highest weight. When a person eats less and loses weight, the body reads that as a survival threat. It has several old, overlapping ways to push its weight back up:[7] metabolism slows, the hormones that signal fullness (like leptin) drop, and the hormones that signal hunger (like ghrelin) rise.[8] These changes can last for years. "Your brain remembers your highest weight," I tell Sarah, "and it wants to take you back there. That's how it thinks it keeps you safe."

She's tried many diets. There were 1,200-calorie meal plans that left her lightheaded in afternoon meetings. The ketogenic diet worked for three months until she couldn't stand the thought of another piece of carb-less bread. Intermittent fasting made her irritable and obsessive. Each time, she lost weight. Each time, the weight came back, often with interest. Each time, she blamed herself.

This is why *eat less, move more* fails for most patients with obesity. It asks the conscious mind to override an involuntary system that regulates hunger and metabolism, and to do that forever. For most people, that isn't sustainable. The willpower required is superhuman, yet we act as if it's reasonable to expect people to stay hungry for life.

The population eligible for anti-obesity medication in the United States is not a niche group. Based on U.S. Food and Drug Administration (FDA) guidelines, individuals with a BMI of 30 or higher (obesity) or 27 or higher (overweight) with at least one weight-related condition qualify for treatment.[9] That's 126 million people. Nearly half the adult population in the United States.

A NEW CLASS OF MEDICINE

Into this landscape of biological resistance and massive unmet need arrived a category-creating class of medications: the glucagon-like peptide-1 receptor agonists, known as 'GLP-1s'.

To understand how they work, you need to know about the incretin effect. In the 1960s and 1970s, researchers observed something curious: glucose taken by mouth triggered a much bigger insulin response than the same amount of glucose given intravenously.[10] This meant the gut was not a passive tube. It was an active endocrine organ. When nutrients enter the digestive tract, they trigger the release of incretin hormones, which signal the pancreas to prepare for incoming energy.

Two hormones mediate this effect: glucose-dependent insulinotropic polypeptide (GIP) and GLP-1. Together, they account for up to 70% of the insulin released after a meal in healthy people. In patients with Type 2 diabetes and obesity, this system is impaired.[11]

The pharmacological challenge was to create molecules that mimic these hormones but remain in the body long enough to be effective as drugs. Native GLP-1 has a half-life of less than two minutes. It is rapidly broken down by the enzyme dipeptidyl peptidase-4 (DPP-4).[12] To create a viable drug, biochemists modified the peptide structure to resist that breakdown and bind to blood albumin, extending its activity from minutes to days.[13]

"We're adding GLP-1 to what your body already releases after a meal," I explain to Sarah. "It tightens the connection between your brain and your gut so your appetite is less intense."

The first generation of these long-acting agents included liraglutide (marketed as Saxenda for obesity). Liraglutide required daily injections and resulted in a modest weight loss of approximately 5-8%.[14] Clinically relevant, but not enough to reshape the obesity treatment landscape.

Everything changed with semaglutide. By substituting specific amino acids in the peptide chain, Novo Nordisk created a molecule that enabled once-weekly dosing and far greater efficacy. Semaglutide corrects several problems at once. It stimulates insulin release in a glucose-dependent way: the pancreas responds to a meal as the stomach breaks it down. As appetite drops and food intake falls, fewer carbohydrates in the meal mean less insulin is needed. It lowers glucagon, the hormone that signals the release of stored fuel. It slows gastric emptying, keeping food in the upper gut longer.[15]

The most important action, though, happens in the brain. Semaglutide reaches the hypothalamus and the brain stem, the command centers for appetite and satiety. It stimulates neurons that signal fullness. It blocks neurons that signal hunger.[16]

Patients describe the effect as the silencing of *food noise*—the constant, intrusive, obsessive thoughts about food that plague many people living with obesity.[17] For the first time, they feel satisfied after a smaller portion. They stop thinking about their next meal while eating their current one.

In the STEP 1 trial, semaglutide 2.4 mg (sold now under the brand name Wegovy) produced a mean weight reduction of 14.9% over 68 weeks.[18] That is roughly three times what legacy anti-obesity medications delivered.[19]

Sarah starts semaglutide at our next appointment. We begin at 0.25 mg weekly.

Twincretin

Then came tirzepatide. If semaglutide defines the category, tirzepatide is the next major leap. Tirzepatide, which is branded as Zepbound for obesity and Mounjaro for diabetes, is a *twincretin*. It is a single peptide that activates receptors for both GLP-1 and GIP.[20]

This was counterintuitive. GIP was historically understood to promote fat storage. But Eli Lilly's scientists discovered that when GIP is combined with GLP-1, it improves insulin sensitivity while reducing some of the nausea associated with GLP-1 alone.[21] GIP receptors are also found in fat tissue, where they appear to help keep fats out of the bloodstream. In the SURMOUNT-1 trial, the highest dose of tirzepatide achieved a mean weight reduction of 20.9% at 72 weeks.[22] In a head-to-head comparison, tirzepatide showed greater weight loss than semaglutide.[23]

We are now seeing weight-loss outcomes from pharmacotherapy that rival bariatric surgery, without the operative risk. For decades, surgery was the only intervention that could reliably produce this magnitude of weight loss. The surgery requires anesthesia, surgical teams, and operating rooms, and it carries a meaningful risk of complications. Now, a once-weekly injection achieves similar outcomes. In my practice, I see patients who were told a decade ago that surgery was their only option. Today, they take a weekly injection and never need the operating room.

Pan-Metabolic Therapy

The value of these medications extends far beyond weight loss. GLP-1 receptors are expressed in the pancreas, heart, kidneys, liver, and lungs. These drugs function as pan-metabolic therapies.[24]

The SELECT trial showed that semaglutide reduced the risk of major cardiovascular events, like heart attack, stroke, and cardiovascular death, by 20% in adults with obesity and heart disease, independent of diabetes status.[25] The FLOW trial showed that semaglutide significantly reduced the risk of kidney failure and death from kidney causes in patients with Type 2 diabetes and chronic kidney disease.[26] Tirzepatide has been shown to reduce the severity of obstructive sleep apnea by up to 63%.[27] Data from the ESSENCE trial show these agents can resolve fatty liver disease and improve liver fibrosis.[28]

One medication can now simultaneously address the clinical priorities of endocrinologists, cardiologists, nephrologists, hepatologists, sleep specialists, and, likely soon, rheumatologists and orthopedic surgeons. This versatility transforms the total addressable market from *patients who want to lose weight* to *patients with any metabolic dysfunction or inflammation.*

What Comes Next

The innovation cycle is accelerating. Retatrutide is a triple agonist targeting GLP-1, GIP, and glucagon receptors. Glucagon agonism increases energy expenditure and suppresses appetite. Phase 2 data showed weight loss of up to 24.2% at 48 weeks.[29] Eli Lilly's orforglipron, launched in 2026, is the first non-peptide, small-molecule oral GLP-1 agonist on the market. It can be manufactured more cheaply than injectable peptides and removes the barriers of injections and cold-chain storage.[30] CagriSema combines semaglutide with cagrilintide, a long-acting amylin analog. Early trial data showed that 29.4% of participants with obesity and type 2 diabetes lost 20% or more of their body weight.[31]

These medications are no longer the rate limiter. They are safe, effective, and capable of reversing the most expensive chronic diseases in the industrialized world.

The Tolerability Trade-Off

There is a trade-off to efficacy. The same mechanisms that make these drugs work by slowing gastric emptying and altering brain signaling may also cause side effects. Patients commonly experience nausea, vomiting, diarrhea, and constipation, particularly during early treatment.[32] For most patients, these effects are mild to moderate and resolve within weeks. For some, they are severe enough to stop treatment.

Early drop-off is common, especially for people with obesity and without diabetes. One industry-funded study of U.S. commercial insurance records found that approximately 30% of patients stop treatment within the first four weeks.[33] A 2024 U.S. study reviewed the records of 195,000 people on GLP-1 medications who had diabetes, obesity, or both.[34] Within 90 days, 35.8% of people with obesity alone had discontinued treatment. By one year, half had stopped taking the medication entirely.

All GLP-1-containing medications carry the FDA's most serious drug safety warning due to a potential association with thyroid C-cell tumors observed in rodent studies, and there is also a slightly elevated risk of pancreatitis and gastroparesis.[35]

The clinical reality is that, although the drugs work, taking them is not easy. Patients need a lot of support to feel well during treatment. When support is missing, patients quit.

At week two, Sarah asks whether we can accelerate her dose-increase schedule. "This is not the Olympics," I tell her. "Faster, higher, stronger dosing is not going to give you more weight loss now. You have to give your body and brain time to adjust." Every step up in dose is a fresh round of side effects. The goal is the lowest dose that gently moderates appetite, leads to sustainable weight loss or maintenance, and is comfortably tolerated.

LIFELONG TREATMENT

The most critical misunderstanding in the current market is the belief that these medications are short-term interventions. They are not. Obesity is a chronic, relapsing disease. There is no cure, only management. A patient who takes semaglutide for six months, loses 30 pounds, and then stops is not cured; she is unmedicated for her condition.

The evidence is unequivocal; when treatment stops, weight returns. In the STEP 1 trial extension, participants who stopped semaglutide regained two-thirds of their lost weight within one year.[36] Blood pressure and blood sugar both rose again. The clinical benefit evaporated (see Figure 1.1).

This is the nature of obesity treatment without maintenance. The body's counter-regulatory mechanisms do not sleep. If the pharmacological brake is removed, the physiological drive to regain weight reasserts itself.[37] Weight regain is the most common predictor of whether a patient will restart therapy.[38] Patients stop, regain, and restart. The cycle destroys clinical value because the patient spends months in a state of uncontrolled disease. Economic value is destroyed because the cost of reacquisition and re-titration is high.

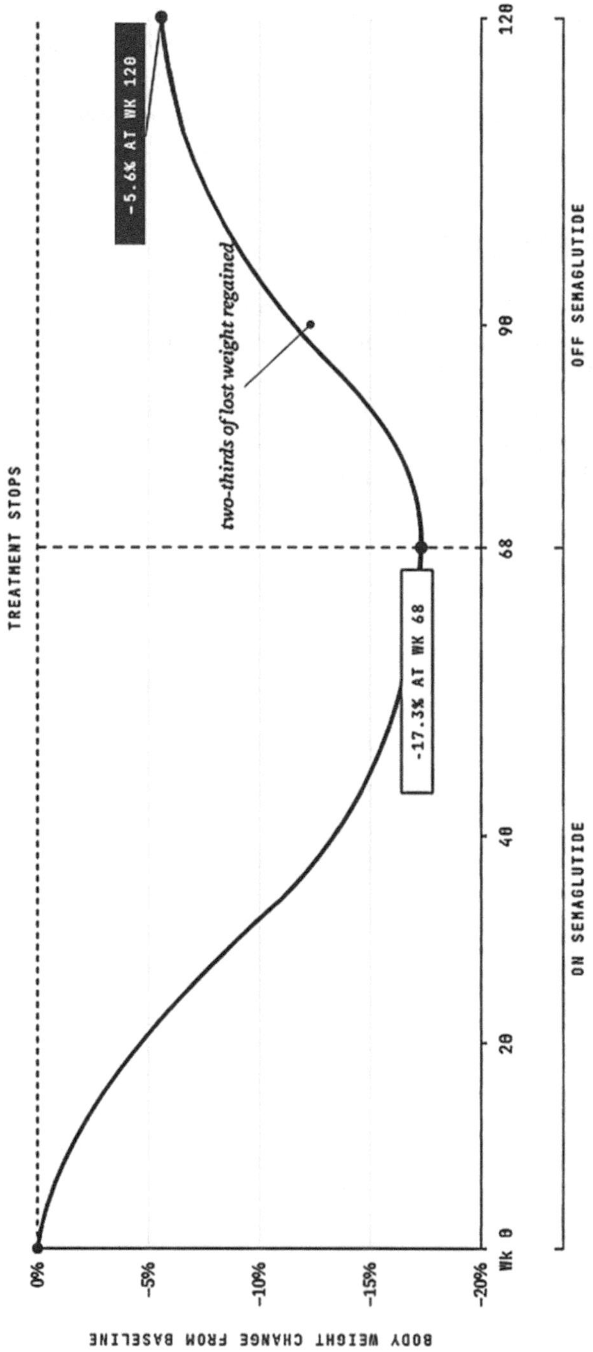

Figure 1.1 When semaglutide is stopped, the weight comes back.

We do not treat high blood pressure for six months, then stop treatment when blood pressure normalizes. We do not treat high cholesterol until low-density lipoprotein (LDL) levels drop, then withdraw the statin. Unless, of course, we manage to solve the underlying root cause of the disease. In many cases, that root cause is obesity.

THE SYSTEM FAILURE

This generation of obesity medications is a triumph of science. It offers patients like Sarah a biological explanation for their struggles and an effective pharmacological solution. Yet we are delivering treatment to only a small fraction of those who need it. Two-thirds of patients discontinue treatment within a year.[39] The gap between what these drugs can do and how they are being delivered is not just a market failure. It is a public health crisis.

ENDNOTES

1. Alison Fildes et al., "Probability of an Obese Person Attaining Normal Body Weight: Cohort Study Using Electronic Health Records," *American Journal of Public Health* 105, no. 9 (2015): e54–59, https://doi.org/10.2105/AJPH.2015.302773.
2. Bryan Stierman et al., "National Health and Nutrition Examination Survey 2017–March 2020 Prepandemic Data Files—Development of Files and Prevalence Estimates for Selected Health Outcomes," in *National Health Statistics Reports* (National Center for Health Statistics (U.S.), 2021), https://doi.org/10.15620/cdc:106273.
3. Zachary J. Ward et al., "Association of Body Mass Index with Health Care Expenditures in the United States by Age and Sex," *PloS One* 16, no. 3 (2021): e0247307, https://doi.org/10.1371/journal.pone.0247307.
4. "9 Promising Obesity Drugs Set to Launch by 2030," *DelveInsight*, May 12, 2025, https://www.delveinsight.com/blog/obesity-drugs-launch.
5. Ania M. Jastreboff et al., "Tirzepatide Once Weekly for the Treatment of Obesity," *New England Journal of Medicine* 387, no. 3 (2022): 205–16, https://doi.org/10.1056/NEJMoa2206038.
6. Chiadi E. Ndumele et al., "A Synopsis of the Evidence for the Science and Clinical Management of Cardiovascular-Kidney-Metabolic (CKM) Syndrome: A Scientific Statement From the American Heart Association," *Circulation* 148, no. 20 (2023): 1636–64, https://doi.org/10.1161/CIR.0000000000001186.
7. Kevin D. Hall and Scott Kahan, "Maintenance of Lost Weight and Long-Term Management of Obesity," *The Medical Clinics of North America* 102, no. 1 (2018): 183–97, https://doi.org/10.1016/j.mcna.2017.08.012.
8. Priya Sumithran et al., "Long-Term Persistence of Hormonal Adaptations to Weight Loss," *New England Journal of Medicine* 365, no. 17 (2011): 1597–604, https://doi.org/10.1056/NEJMI105816.
9. Jennifer H. Hwang et al., "Lifetime Health Effects and Cost-Effectiveness of Tirzepatide and Semaglutide in U.S. Adults," *JAMA Health Forum* 6, no. 3 (2025): e245586, https://doi.org/10.1001/jamahealthforum.2024.5586.
10. Qiyuan Keith Liu, "Mechanisms of Action and Therapeutic Applications of GLP-1 and Dual GIP/GLP-1 Receptor Agonists," *Frontiers in Endocrinology* 15 (July 2024), https://doi.org/10.3389/fendo.2024.1431292.
11. Laurie L. Baggio and Daniel J. Drucker, "Biology of Incretins: GLP-1 and GIP," *Gastroenterology* 132, no. 6 (2007): 2131–57, https://doi.org/10.1053/j.gastro.2007.03.054.
12. Carolyn F. Deacon et al., "Both Subcutaneously and Intravenously Administered Glucagon-Like Peptide I Are Rapidly Degraded From the NH2-Terminus in Type II Diabetic Patients and in Healthy Subjects," *Diabetes* 44, no. 9 (1995): 1126–31, https://doi.org/10.2337/diab.44.9.1126.
13. Liu, "Mechanisms of Action and Therapeutic Applications of GLP-1 and Dual GIP/GLP-1 Receptor Agonists."

14. Young Jin Tak and Sang Yeoup Lee, "Long-Term Efficacy and Safety of Anti-Obesity Treatment: Where Do We Stand?," *Current Obesity Reports* 10, no. 1 (2021): 14–30, https://doi.org/10.1007/s13679-020-00422-w.
15. Daniel J. Drucker, "Mechanisms of Action and Therapeutic Application of Glucagon-like Peptide-1," *Cell Metabolism* 27, no. 4 (2018): 740–56, https://doi.org/10.1016/j.cmet.2018.03.001.
16. Drucker, "Mechanisms of Action and Therapeutic Application of Glucagon-like Peptide-1."
17. Emily J. Dhurandhar et al., "Food Noise: Definition, Measurement, and Future Research Directions," *Nutrition & Diabetes* 15 (2025): 30, https://doi.org/10.1038/s41387-025-00382-x.
18. John P. H. Wilding et al., "Once-Weekly Semaglutide in Adults with Overweight or Obesity," *New England Journal of Medicine* 384, no. 11 (2021): 989–1002, https://doi.org/10.1056/NEJMoa2032183.
19. Tak and Lee, "Long-Term Efficacy and Safety of Anti-Obesity Treatment."
20. Julio Rosenstock et al., "Efficacy and Safety of a Novel Dual GIP and GLP-1 Receptor Agonist Tirzepatide in Patients with Type 2 Diabetes (SURPASS-1): A Double-Blind, Randomised, Phase 3 Trial," *The Lancet* 398, no. 10295 (2021): 143–55, https://doi.org/10.1016/S0140-6736(21)01324-6.
21. Ricardo J. Samms et al., "How May GIP Enhance the Therapeutic Efficacy of GLP-1?," *Trends in Endocrinology and Metabolism: TEM* 31, no. 6 (2020): 410–21, https://doi.org/10.1016/j.tem.2020.02.006.
22. Jastreboff et al., "Tirzepatide Once Weekly for the Treatment of Obesity."
23. Patricia J. Rodriguez et al., "Semaglutide vs Tirzepatide for Weight Loss in Adults With Overweight or Obesity," *JAMA Internal Medicine* 184, no. 9 (2024): 1056–64, https://doi.org/10.1001/jamainternmed.2024.2525.
24. Liu, "Mechanisms of Action and Therapeutic Applications of GLP-1 and Dual GIP/GLP-1 Receptor Agonists."
25. A. Michael Lincoff et al., "Semaglutide and Cardiovascular Outcomes in Obesity without Diabetes," *New England Journal of Medicine* 389, no. 24 (2023): 2221–32, https://doi.org/10.1056/NEJMoa2307563.
26. Vlado Perkovic et al., "Effects of Semaglutide on Chronic Kidney Disease in Patients with Type 2 Diabetes," *New England Journal of Medicine* 391, no. 2 (2024): 109–21, https://doi.org/10.1056/NEJMoa2403347.
27. Atul Malhotra et al., "Tirzepatide for the Treatment of Obstructive Sleep Apnea and Obesity," *New England Journal of Medicine* 391, no. 13 (2024): 1193–205, https://doi.org/10.1056/NEJMoa2404881.
28. Arun J. Sanyal et al., "Phase 3 Trial of Semaglutide in Metabolic Dysfunction-Associated Steatohepatitis," *The New England Journal of Medicine* 392, no. 21 (2025): 2089–99, https://doi.org/10.1056/NEJMoa2413258.
29. "9 Promising Obesity Drugs Set to Launch by 2030," *DelveInsight*, May 12, 2025, https://www.delveinsight.com/blog/obesity-drugs-launch.

30. "Eli Lilly Knockout Quarter Beat and Raise Widens the Lead," October 30, 2025, https://www.home.saxo/content/articles/equities/eli-lilly-knockout-quarter-beat-and-raise-widens-the-lead-30102025.
31. Daniel J. Drucker, "The Expanding Landscape of GLP-1 Medicines," *Nature Medicine*, ahead of print, January 2, 2026, https://doi.org/10.1038/s41591-025-04124-5.
32. Mohit Sodhi et al., "Risk of Gastrointestinal Adverse Events Associated With Glucagon-Like Peptide-1 Receptor Agonists for Weight Loss," *JAMA* 330, no. 18 (2023): 1795–97, https://doi.org/10.1001/jama.2023.19574.
33. Blue Health Intelligence, *Real-World Trends in GLP-1 Treatment Persistence and Prescribing for Weight Management* (Blue Health Intelligence, 2024).
34. Duy Do et al., "GLP-1 Receptor Agonist Discontinuation Among Patients With Obesity and/or Type 2 Diabetes," *JAMA Network Open* 7, no. 5 (2024): e2413172, https://doi.org/10.1001/jamanetworkopen.2024.13172.
35. *Wegovy (Semaglutide) Injection, for Subcutaneous Use: Prescribing Information*, Reference ID: 4806455 (U.S. Food and Drug Administration, 2021), 34.
36. John P. H. Wilding et al., "Weight Regain and Cardiometabolic Effects after Withdrawal of Semaglutide: The STEP 1 Trial Extension," *Diabetes, Obesity & Metabolism* 24, no. 8 (2022): 1553–64, https://doi.org/10.1111/dom.14725.
37. Kevin D. Hall, "Physiology of the Weight-Loss Plateau in Response to Diet Restriction, GLP-1 Receptor Agonism, and Bariatric Surgery," *Obesity (Silver Spring, Md.)* 32, no. 6 (2024): 1163–68, https://doi.org/10.1002/oby.24027.
38. Patricia J. Rodriguez et al., "Discontinuation and Reinitiation of Dual-Labeled GLP-1 Receptor Agonists Among U.S. Adults With Overweight or Obesity," *JAMA Network Open* 8, no. 1 (2025): e2457349, https://doi.org/10.1001/jamanetworkopen.2024.57349.
39. Rodriguez et al., "Discontinuation and Reinitiation of Dual-Labeled GLP-1 Receptor Agonists Among U.S. Adults With Overweight or Obesity."

CHAPTER 2

THE MONETIZATION OF OBESITY MEDICINE

Sarah comes back six weeks after starting semaglutide. She has lost five pounds. "I can hear myself think now. I want to eat, and then I can stop without a whole drama taking place in my head. And then I don't think about it again until it's time for my next meal!" She is also sleeping better and has less knee pain. For the first time in 20 years, she feels like her body makes sense. Sarah is one of the lucky ones. She has insurance that covers the medication. She has a copay she can afford. She found a clinic that can prescribe these drugs and support patients through their side effects.

THE MARKET GAP

If you look at sales data for the brand-name obesity medications (e.g., Wegovy and Zepbound) and for the diabetes brands (e.g., Ozempic and Mounjaro) used by people without diabetes, the U.S. market reached 3.4% of its total in 2025.[1] Something is broken in obesity medicine. We have drugs that work really well. We have manufacturers who have invested over $50 billion *each* in factory capacity to make enough medication for everyone who needs it.[2] There are around 126 million Americans who meet the clinical criteria for treatment.[3]

The 126 million figure comes from a 2025 *JAMA Health Forum* analysis by Hwang and colleagues, which modeled U.S. Centers for Disease Control and Prevention (CDC) data against eligibility criteria for obesity medications: a body mass index (BMI) of 30 or higher, the clinical threshold for obesity, or a BMI of 27 or higher combined with at least one weight-related disease.[4] This is about 47% of U.S. adults aged 20 to 79, or roughly half the country. The CDC's separate prevalence figures point in the same direction. More than 40% of U.S. adults have obesity, and a meaningful share of the additional 31% in the overweight range carry at least one qualifying illness.

Of the 126 million eligible adults, many will never end up on a GLP-1. Some do not want to lose weight. Others will not take a weekly injection for the rest of their life. Medical contraindications and specific intolerances exclude others. The 126 million figure also excludes a portion of the population it should include. As approved indications expand into cardiovascular risk reduction, kidney disease, obstructive sleep apnea, and metabolic liver disease, adults who carry one of these conditions but fall outside the BMI eligibility criteria become eligible. For the calculations that follow, I anchor on 126 million as a working figure.

Defining the Gap

Before we can measure how much money is being left on the table, we need a common vocabulary. The theoretical maximum market size is calculated by multiplying the number of people who could be treated by the cost of treating them for a year. This is the *total addressable market* (TAM). For obesity medications, that is 126 million eligible patients multiplied by the average *annual treatment cost* (ATC). Nobody expects to capture TAM. It is the ceiling on the market.

Inside TAM sits a smaller piece: the people the system can actually reach right now. This accounts for insurance coverage, prescriber availability, whether the drugs are included on special pharmacy lists called formularies, and whether a patient even knows these drugs exist. This is the *serviceable available market* (SAM). SAM tells you what is achievable if every market factor is optimized.

The *serviceable obtainable market* (SOM) factors in competition, production capacity, and marketing effectiveness. SOM is what companies are going for in their annual plans. Then there is *actual revenue*, which is the income companies actually earn. The gap between actual revenue and a reasonable SOM is the money being left on the table. In obesity medicine, that gap is perplexing (see Figure 2.1).

A WARNING FROM ANOTHER DRUG CLASS

Before we calculate the gap, it is worth examining how other breakthrough chronic-disease medications have performed. Jardiance, Farxiga, and Invokana[5] are medications to treat type 2 diabetes and are also approved for heart failure and kidney disease. They work by blocking a protein that absorbs glucose and sodium into the bloodstream. This class of medications is known as SGLT2 (sodium-glucose cotransporter-2) inhibitors.

SGLT2 inhibitors look like GLP-1 medications on paper. Both treat chronic diseases within large, stable patient populations. Both require maintenance therapy with high renewal potential. Both have expanded from diabetes into cardio-renal indications. Both carry strong guideline endorsement and broad payer coverage.[6]

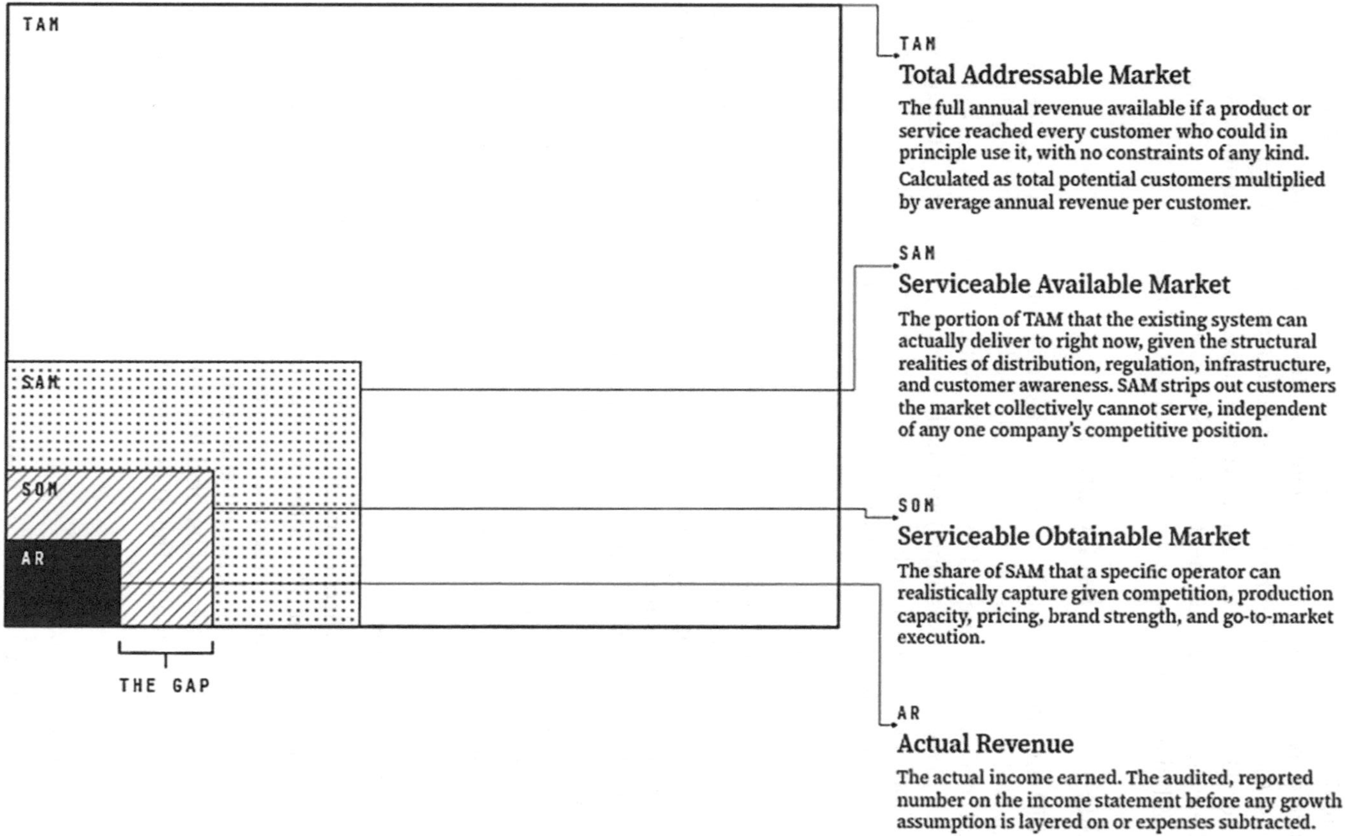

Figure 2.1 Defining the market gap. *Source*: Bill Aulet, Disciplined Entrepreneurship: 24 Steps to a Successful Startup, exp. and updated 2nd ed. Hoboken, NJ: Wiley, 2024.

SGLT2 inhibitors also lack the stigma that has historically constrained obesity drugs. There are no major coverage exclusions, unlike obesity medications.

In 2024, the U.S. SGLT2 inhibitor market generated approximately $6.6 billion in revenue.[7] The number of U.S. adults with diagnosed type 2 diabetes was 26 million.[8] The average annual treatment cost for SGLT2 inhibitors was $3,500, giving a TAM of $91 billion. The class captured 7.3% of its total market.

Why GLP-1s Should Be Different

The SGLT2 inhibitors establish a baseline trajectory for a hero drug class that is fully endorsed by medical specialty organizations, has a decade of safety data, and has broad coverage by insurers. The floor is 7%. But GLP-1 medications like semaglutide (e.g., Wegovy and Ozempic) and dual-agonist medications like tirzepatide (e.g., Zepbound and Mounjaro) have structural advantages over SGLT2 inhibitors. The bar for success is much higher than for SGLT2 inhibitors.

1. Appetite Advantage

These medications target the hypothalamus, the brain's metabolic command center.[9] This is where the appetite originates.[10] By activating satiety neurons in the brain, GLP-1s and dual-agonist medications address appetite at its source. Patients eat less, feel satisfied, and stop obsessing about food between meals.

SGLT2 inhibitors only work downstream. They stop glucose reabsorption in the kidney and force excretion of 60 to 80 grams of glucose per day.[11] But they do nothing to the hormonal drivers of eating. GLP-1s make patients want less. SGLT2 inhibitors help dispose of what has already been consumed. The difference matters because wanting less food makes weight loss easier. Patients on SGLT2 inhibitors must still regulate their appetite every day.

2. Positive Reinforcement

Weight loss is visible.[12] When a patient loses 15% of their body weight, everyone notices. The mirror shows it. The clothes display it. The comments at work confirm it. For better and worse, the transformation is public. SGLT2 inhibitor efficacy, by contrast, hides in lab values. A patient may see improved HbA1c or stable kidney function, which is clinically vital but invisible where the patient lives, works, and interacts with their community. The GLP-1 class should be winning on psychology alone.

3. Pan-Metabolic Treatment

SGLT2 receptors are found almost exclusively in the kidneys. As Chapter 1 established, GLP-1 receptors are distributed throughout the body. Wide receptor distribution opened the door to label expansion into cardiovascular risk reduction, obstructive sleep apnea, metabolic liver disease, osteoarthritis, and potentially neurodegeneration.[13] The SURMOUNT-OSA trial showed tirzepatide reduced sleep apnea severity by up to 63%.[14] The ESSENCE trial demonstrated that semaglutide could resolve the fatty infiltration of the liver in 63% of patients with metabolic liver disease.[15] Multiple benefits mean multiple revenue streams for the same medication.

4. Culture Craze

GLP-1 medications have achieved viral cultural relevance: #ozempic has garnered hundreds of millions of views on social media. Influencers and celebrities document their journeys publicly.[16] Patients now arrive in my office asking specifically for *the weight loss shot*. The adoption of SGLT2 inhibitors depends on physicians to initiate their use. GLP-1s have cultural tailwinds that should translate directly to better market capture.

5. Market Size

There are over one billion people living with obesity globally, with an additional 1.5 billion whose BMI falls in the overweight range. The obesity market had no meaningful pharmacological competition until the arrival of semaglutide. The only alternative was bariatric surgery. Meanwhile, SGLT2 inhibitors compete with metformin, sulfonylureas, DPP-4 inhibitors, and insulin. A first-mover class in a vastly larger market, with zero generic competition, should be capturing far more than a mature class fighting for placement in a commoditized category.

WHAT THESE MEDICATIONS ACTUALLY COST

List prices for medications are fictional in the United States. When Wegovy's sticker reads $1,349 per month, that number obscures the economics of the market. Discounts, rebates, and fees accumulate between the factory and the pharmacy. The gap between list price and actual price realized by the manufacturer ranges from 24% to 73%.[17]

To understand why, meet the middlemen. They are called pharmacy benefit managers (PBMs). Think of a PBM as the broker between the drug company and your insurance plan. They were created to negotiate prices on behalf of insurers and employers. In practice, they have become extraction machines.

Here is how it works: a drug company sets a list price of $1,000. The PBM goes to the drug company and says, "Give us a $600 rebate, and we will put your drug on our preferred list." The drug company agrees because without preferred placement, insurers will not cover the medication, and doctors will not write the prescription. The PBM then charges the employer $900 for the drug, pays the pharmacy $700, and keeps the spread. The patient's copay is calculated using the $1,000 list price, not the $400 the PBM actually paid. The patient pays more. The employer pays more. The PBM keeps the difference.

Mark Cuban, who built a company called Cost Plus Drugs to bypass this exact problem, describes the mechanism bluntly. In a 2025 interview, he characterized the U.S. healthcare system as a $4.9 trillion pool in which "*wherever anybody can arbitrage whatever they can out of the system, that is exactly what they are going to do.*"[18] Cuban calls it *financial engineering disguised as healthcare administration.* Complexity is the product, and opacity enables arbitrage. Nobody knows what anything costs. Everyone is paying more than they should.

The metric that matters is the average ATC. That is the net revenue after all the middlemen take their cuts. It is what manufacturers actually receive.

Semaglutide (Wegovy and Ozempic)

In 2024, the U.S. list price for Wegovy was $1,349 per month, or about $16,200 per year.[19] But the net realized price per patient was significantly lower, approximately $650 per month, or $7,788 per year.[20] Independent evaluations by the Institute for Clinical and Economic Review (ICER) landed in a similar range.[21]

The clinical story strengthened the economic case for insurance coverage. When semaglutide earned a cardiovascular risk-reduction indication, payer approval rates in Medicare Part D jumped from 12% to 20% in a single year.[22] The drug transitioned from being seen as a *weight-loss* drug to a *cardiovascular* drug—a framing shift that bypassed historical Medicare prohibitions on covering obesity medications.[23]

Tirzepatide (Zepbound and Mounjaro)

Eli Lilly entered the market with an aggressive pricing strategy designed to undercut Wegovy. Zepbound's list price was set at roughly $1,060 per month, or about $12,700 per year.[24] The ATC in 2024 was estimated at $7,973 per year.[25]

Eli Lilly understood that as prices decreased, prescription volume would increase. Zepbound sales tripled in 2025 to over $9 billion.[26] By launching LillyDirect pricing at $349 per month for starter doses, the company established a secondary price floor for the uninsured and began learning how to sell at scale.[27] The program operates through partner telehealth companies for prescribing and through separate fulfillment channels for distribution, while demonstrating a key point: patients will pay out of pocket when prices reach accessible levels.

WHY 15% IS CONSERVATIVE, NOT ASPIRATIONAL

Throughout this analysis, I use 15% market penetration as the benchmark for what should be achievable. This number is not aspirational. It is grounded in peer-reviewed health-economic modeling and validated by federal budget projections.

In 2020, researchers published a landmark study in *Obesity* that modeled the societal value of expanding access to anti-obesity medications.[28] At that time, these drugs were prescribed to fewer than 2% of eligible patients. The authors chose a 15% uptake specifically to simulate *modest* expansion—not universal coverage; not aggressive adoption; just a reasonable increase from the negligible baseline for an important disease. They found that even this limited improvement would generate an estimated $1.2 trillion in societal value through reduced medical costs, decreased disability, and gains in quality-adjusted life-years.[29]

The 15% figure was deliberately conservative. The same researchers contrasted it with a 30% scenario designed to model what might happen with Wegovy and Zepbound, which had not yet reached the market.[30] In other words, the 15% benchmark was calibrated to older, less effective medications. With drugs now demonstrating 15% to 22% weight loss rather than 5% to 7%, the case for achieving 15% penetration is stronger, not weaker.

Federal projections now validate this benchmark. In October 2024, the Congressional Budget Office estimated that if Medicare authorized coverage for obesity medications, take-up would rise from 2% in 2026 to 14% by 2034.[31] The gap calculations that follow use this benchmark not as a fantasy of what could be, but as a defensible estimate of what should be.

The Gap: 2024

Let's start with the revenue. The U.S. sales of obesity medications,[32] including Wegovy and Zepbound, totaled approximately $11.7 billion in 2024.[33] These are known as *on-label* sales. But these medications are also prescribed *off-label* for weight loss to patients without diabetes. That off-label revenue, primarily from Ozempic and Mounjaro, added another $7.8 billion.[34] When you combine the on-label and off-label sales, the estimated total annual revenue for these medications for weight loss in the United States was $19.5 billion.

At the 2024 ATC of $7,880 per patient, the theoretical ceiling is 126 million eligible adults multiplied by that cost: roughly $992.9 billion. Against actual revenue of $19.5 billion, the industry captured less than 2% of the theoretical market (see Figure 2.2).

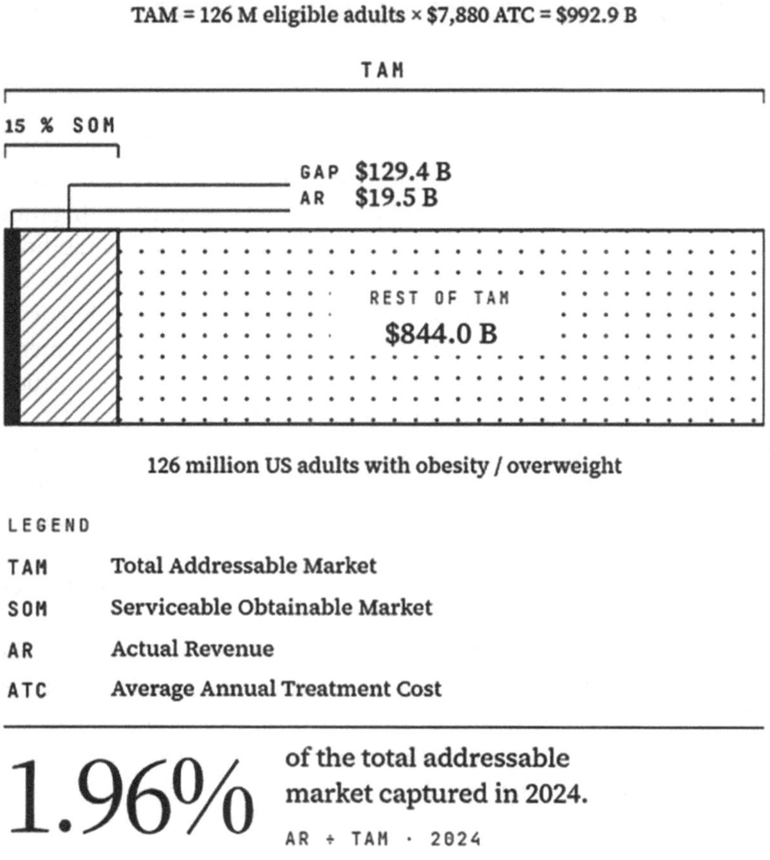

Figure 2.2 The 2024 U.S. obesity medication market.

Sources: Novo Nordisk A/S, Financial Report for the Period 1 January 2024 to 31 December 2024, Form 6-K (Washington, DC: U.S. Securities and Exchange Commission, February 5, 2025), https://www.sec.gov/Archives/edgar/data/353278/000162828025003924/caq42024.htm; Eli Lilly and Company, "Lilly Reports Full Q4 2024 Financial Results and Provides 2025 Guidance," news release, February 6, 2025, https://investor.lilly.com/news-releases/news-release-details/lilly-reports-full-q4-2024-financial-results-and-provides-2025. Author's calculation; Off-label proportion derived from Kateri J. Spinelli et al., "Health Disparity Clusters of Off Label Prescriptions for Glucagon-Like Peptide 1 Receptor Agonists," *American Journal of Medicine Open* 13 (June 2025): 100100, https://doi.org/10.1016/j.ajmo.2025.100100, which found a median off-label rate of 37.7% in a 2022 all-payer dataset of 3,688,430 prescriptions for type-2-diabetes-indicated GLP-1 RAs. Applied to 2024 U.S. Ozempic and Mounjaro net revenue derived from Novo Nordisk's Form 6-K (FY2024) and Eli Lilly's Q4 2024 earnings release.

Here's the math:

Theoretical TAM: 126 million eligible adults × $7,880 = **$992.9 billion**
Actual revenue: $19.5 billion
Market capture rate: 1.96%

But TAM is an impossible abstraction. The number that matters is the 15% benchmark that health economists consider achievable:

15% SOM: 18.9 million patients × $7,880 = **$148.9 billion**
2024 Gap (15% SOM vs. actual revenue): $148.9B – $19.5B = **$129.4 billion**

A note on these numbers: Each input carries a margin of error. The off-label revenue allocation of 38% is most accurate for 2024 but likely went down as on-label treatments became more available in 2026. The $7,880 ATC is my calculated weighted average across products, channels, and negotiated rates.

In 2024, the industry left nearly $130 billion on the table compared to what conservative health-economic modeling suggests is achievable. Given the margins of error, consider the calculated gaps for 2024, 2025, and 2026 directional based on the best publicly available data. The directionality is what matters when understanding this market.

The Gap: 2025

In 2025, Wegovy generated approximately $7.5 billion in U.S. revenue,[35] while Zepbound generated $13.54 billion.[36] The off-label revenue added approximately $10.34 billion.[37,38,39] The total revenue for the U.S. obesity pharmacotherapy market in 2025 was $31.4 billion, as shown in Figure 2.3.

At the 2025 ATC of $7,401:[40]

Theoretical TAM: 126 million × $7,401 = **$932.5 billion**
Actual revenue: $31.4 billion
Market capture rate: 3.37%
15% SOM: $139.9 billion
2025 Gap (15% SOM vs. actual revenue): $139.9B – S31.4B = **$108.5 billion**

Progress. The market capture rate only rose from just under 2% to nearly 3.4%. But the gap, the distance between where we are and where health economists say we should be, remained over $100 billion.

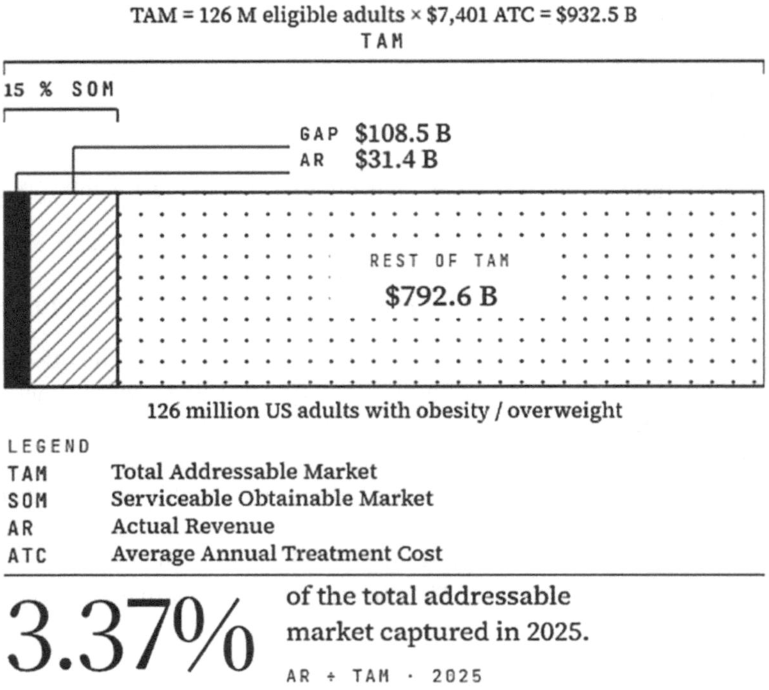

Figure 2.3 The 2025 U.S. obesity medication market.

Sources: Novo Nordisk A/S, Financial Report for the Period 1 January 2025 to 31 December 2025, Form 6-K (Washington, DC: U.S. Securities and Exchange Commission, February 4, 2026), https://www.sec.gov/Archives/edgar/data/353278/000035327826000012/nvo-20251231.htm.; Eli Lilly and Company, Lilly Reports Fourth-Quarter 2025 Financial Results and Provides 2026 Guidance, Form 8-K (Washington, DC: U.S. Securities and Exchange Commission, February 4, 2026), https://www.sec.gov/Archives/edgar/data/0000059478/000005947826000008/q425lillysalesandearningsp.htm.; U.S. Mounjaro figures calculated from quarterly disclosures across Lilly's 2025 Form 8-K releases (Q1 May 1, 2025; Q2 August 7, 2025; Q3 October 30, 2025; Q4 February 4, 2026). Wegovy U.S. Operations sales of DKK 51,015 million, converted to USD at the 2025 industry-conventional rate of approximately 6.8 DKK/USD; U.S. Ozempic and Rybelsus estimated from Novo Nordisk's U.S. Operations GLP-1 diabetes care total, after accounting for declining U.S. sales of Rybelsus and Victoza, as disclosed in the same report; Off-label proportion derived from Kevin J. Spinelli et al., "Health Disparity Clusters of Off Label Prescriptions for Glucagon-Like Peptide 1 Receptor Agonists," *American Journal of Medicine Open* 13 (June 2025): 100100, https://doi.org/10.1016/j.ajmo.2025.100100, which found a median county-level off-label prescribing rate of 37.7% (interquartile range 30.0–46.3%) for GLP-1 receptor agonists approved for type 2 diabetes; rounded to 38% and applied to the off-label-eligible denominator (Ozempic, Mounjaro, Rybelsus); ATC of $7,401 derived from Don Tracy, "ICER Releases Cost Analysis Report on Obesity Treatments Semaglutide, Tirzepatide," Pharmaceutical Commerce, December 22, 2025, https://www.pharmaceuticalcommerce.com/view/icer-releases-cost-analysis-report-obesity-treatments-semaglutide-tirzepatide.

The Gap: 2026

Forecasting 2026 requires a different methodology (see Figure 2.4). I model 2026 based on patient-years, defined as the number of people maintained on continuous treatment throughout the year. Based on the actual revenue and average treatment cost, the U.S. obesity market covered approximately 2.47 million patient-years in 2024 and 4.24 million in 2025.[41]

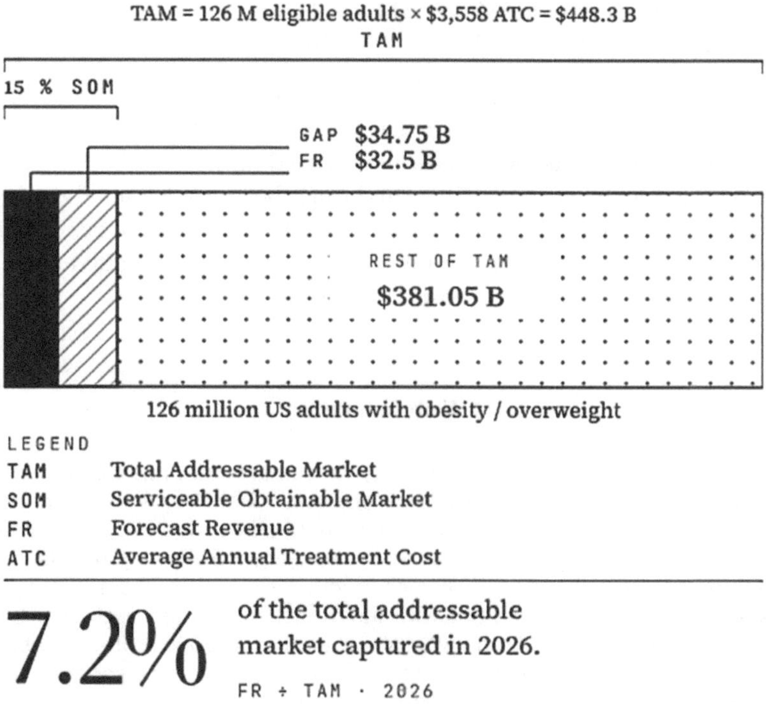

Figure 2.4 The 2026 U.S. obesity medication market.

Sources: ATC: Author's calculation based on estimated mean annual therapy cost derived from negotiated price ranges of $2,940 to $4,200 for Wegovy and $2,940 to $4,152 for Zepbound, yielding an average estimated annual cost of approximately $3,808 per patient. Oral formulations are held out of this scenario modeling because meaningful 2026 sales data do not yet exist. Congressional Budget Office, How Would Authorizing Medicare to Cover Anti-Obesity Medications Affect the Federal Budget?; Pearson et al., "Affordable Access to GLP-1 Obesity Medications"; Wegovy Market Size to Hit USD 24.53 Billion by 2034, no. 6404 (Precedence Research, 2025), https://www.precedenceresearch.com/wegovy-market; House, "Fact Sheet"; Eli Lilly and Company, "Lilly Reports Third-Quarter 2025 Financial Results, Highlights R&D Pipeline Momentum and Raises 2025 Guidance"; Transcribing, "Novo Nordisk (NVO) Q3 2025 Earnings Transcript."

For the 2026 scenario, I use an ATC of $3,558 for Wegovy and Zepbound, the mean of the negotiated price ranges for both medications.[42] This is the most heavily discounted pricing available, and it demonstrates the effect of maximum price compression:

Theoretical TAM: 126M × $3,558 = **$448.3B**
15% SOM: 18.9M × $3,558 = **$67.25B**
Forecast revenue: 9.13M × $3,558 = **$32.5B**
Market capture rate: 126M ÷ 9.13M = **7.2%**
2026 Gap: $67.25B – $32.5B = **$34.75 billion**

If we assume the lowest possible unit prices and significant on-label volume expansion for other diseases, gross U.S. 2026 revenue for on-label Wegovy and Zepbound and off-label Ozempic and Mounjaro is projected at $32.5 billion, representing 7.2% market capture (see Figure 2.5).[43] This brings the forecasted number of person-years treated to 9.13 million, or less than half of the 15% revenue benchmark. For medications with near-universal brand awareness and demonstrated clinical efficacy, something beyond price is constraining expansion.

A Note on Orals

In 2026, the menu expanded. Rybelsus (oral semaglutide) has been marketed since 2019 for the treatment of type 2 diabetes. Oral Wegovy (a higher-dose oral semaglutide formulated for obesity) launched in early 2026, and Eli Lilly's Orforglipron, the first non-peptide small-molecule oral GLP-1 agonist, launched the same year at a reported $349 per month through LillyDirect pricing. The orals are not included in the 2026 revenue model, since meaningful sales data for oral Wegovy and Orforglipron will not exist until mid-2026 at the earliest, and any projection today would be speculation. I treat the orals as a separate thread throughout the book and return to them in Part II.

YEAR	ATC	TAM	SOM AT 15%	AR	MARKET CAPTURE	GAP (15% SOM VS. ACTUAL REVENUE)
2024	$7,880	$992.9 billion	$148.9 billion	$19.5 billion	2.0%	$129.4 billion
2025	$7,401	$932.5 billion	$139.9 billion	$31.4 billion	3.4%	$108.5 billion
2026	$3,558	$448.3 billion	$67.25 billion	FORECAST $32.5 billion	7.2%	$34.75 billion

Figure 2.5 The 2024–2026 obesity medication market size based on a revenue-first analysis. Author's calculations.

WHY MANUFACTURERS MAY ACCEPT LOWER REVENUE

The willingness of Eli Lilly and Novo Nordisk to risk lower revenue in 2026 appears counterintuitive. But manufacturers have built protection mechanisms into their pricing strategy.

The pipeline comes first. The $350 price point applies to current medications, but both companies are preparing to launch superior next-generation drugs at premium prices. Novo Nordisk's CagriSema and Eli Lilly's retatrutide have demonstrated even greater efficacy in trials; retatrutide achieved 24.2% weight loss.[44] Lower prices on current drugs turn them into loss leaders to acquire patients who can later upgrade. Then there is the insurance coverage. Current price concessions apply when the medications are prescribed for obesity or overweight. But both drugs carry approvals for other medical conditions, where coverage is mandatory and reimbursement is higher.[45]

The rebate math also shifts in their favor. In 2025, manufacturers paid rebates of 40% to 60% to PBM for formulary access. Sales through LillyDirect pricing eliminate the PBM rebate entirely.[46] A $1,000 list price minus a $600 rebate yields $400. A $350 direct price with no rebate yields $350. It's nearly all the same for the manufacturer, but they can reach more people.

Contract timing with large insurers also provides a buffer. Contracts lock in for one- to three-year cycles.[47] Many 2026 commercial rates were negotiated at 2024 prices. Plans pay the higher rates even as the cash market drops.

Finally, compounded semaglutide and tirzepatide are easily available on dozens of digital health platforms for $125 to $400 per month.[48] The 2025 financial success of digital health platforms selling compounded GLP-1s has put enormous pressure on drugmakers to lower prices.

Another Slice of the 2025 Data

The previously described market capture approach works backward from the gross revenue of brand-name medications prescribed for weight loss, both on- and off-label. A second approach starts with consumer research on who is taking GLP-1 drugs and reveals just how large the gray market for compounded GLP-1s became in 2025. This is the prevalence-first approach.

Triangulating Prevalence

Three independent U.S. surveys have measured GLP-1 prevalence in the past two years. They tell a fascinating story. The Kaiser Family Foundation (KFF) fielded its first GLP-1 tracking poll in April and May 2024, surveying 1,479 adults and reporting that 12% had ever taken a GLP-1 and 6% were currently taking one.[49] One year later, the RAND Corporation surveyed 8,793 adults from its American Life Panel and reported that 11.8% of U.S. adults had ever taken a GLP-1, with a 95% confidence interval of 10.9% to 12.7%.[50] The data firm Evidation, which you will read more about in Chapter 16, surveyed 109,126 participants; 10% endorsed current or past GLP-1 use.[51] KFF then presented the same questions in October and November 2025 with 1,350 adults. The number of adults currently taking a GLP-1 had doubled to 12%, and the number of adults who had ever taken a GLP-1 had climbed to 18%.[52]

The two KFF polls show the gap between *ever taken* and *currently taking* held steady at six percentage points. In May 2024, the percentages were 12% ever taken and 6% currently taking. In November 2025, the numbers were 18% ever taken and 12% currently taking. The absolute numbers doubled, but leakage stayed the same. Roughly half of every cohort that ever started a GLP-1 is no longer on one. We will use 12% as a measure of current GLP-1 use to estimate the size of the actual 2025 market.

2026 Price Compression

Three things changed sharply between May and November 2025:

1. The U.S. Food and Drug Administration (FDA) declared the semaglutide shortage resolved in February 2025, with compounder grace periods ending in May, though enforcement has been slow to materialize
2. LillyDirect expanded $349 tirzepatide vial pricing throughout 2025

3. TrumpRx negotiations dominated headlines through October and November

The TrumpRx program represents the most significant federal intervention in the pricing of obesity medications to date. Under its negotiated framework, prices dropped fast: Wegovy fell from its list price of $1,350 to about $350 per month. For some Medicare and Medicaid enrollees, the negotiated price was *supposed* to drop further to $245 per month in 2026. This will be discussed in more detail in Chapter 11.[53]

Prevalence-First

Applied to approximately 268 million U.S. adults reported by the Census, the November 2025 KFF figure yields 32.2 million current GLP-1 users across all indications.[54] KFF also reports usage rates by condition. Forty-five percent of adults with diabetes were currently on a GLP-1, and 23% of adults with obesity or overweight in the past five years were currently on a GLP-1.[55] With approximately 29.1 million Americans living with some type of diagnosed diabetes, 13.1 million of the current GLP-1 users do so for diabetes. Of these, the substantial majority have type 2 diabetes and use these medications for both glycemic control and weight loss. There are 19.1 million people who use a GLP-1 but do not have a diabetes diagnosis (see Figure 2.6).[56]

A diabetes diagnosis does not always explain any given patient's rationale for taking a GLP-1. The 29.1 million diagnosed diabetes population includes 1.8 million American adults living with type 1 diabetes. No GLP-1 medication is FDA-approved for type 1 diabetes, but a 2025 analysis showed that by 2023, GLP-1 prescriptions rose to about a third of those with type 1 diabetes who also have severe obesity.[57]

In our earlier analysis, the 2025 actual revenue was $31.4 billion. Divided by the average ATC of $7,401, this covers approximately 4.24 million person-years, assuming all those people remain on treatment throughout the year. To convert person-years to unique persons, we divide by the average duration of therapy. As reported by Duy Do and his colleagues, using the proportion of days covered (PDC) of 54.4% at 12 months for obesity-only GLP-1 patients, there were approximately 7.79 million unique people using branded medication for weight loss in 2025.[58]

Why does the prevalence-first method give us 19.1 million people while the revenue-first method gives us just 7.79 million? Neither number is exact and the inputs are subject to error, as mentioned earlier in this chapter. The 19.1 million comes from the KFF self-reported survey and runs higher than the RAND and

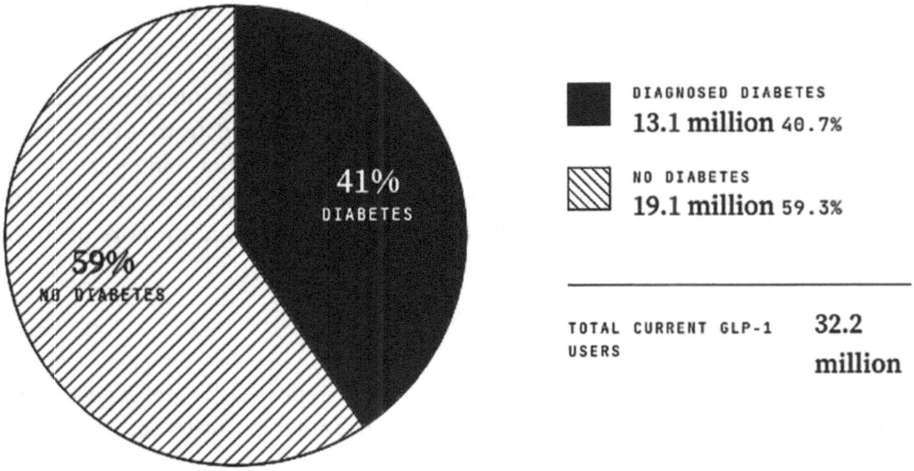

Figure 2.6 Current GLP-1 use by condition.

Sources: Centers for Disease Control and Prevention, "National Diabetes Statistics Report," last updated January 21, 2026, https://www.cdc.gov/diabetes/php/data-research/index.html.; "KFF Health Tracking Poll November 2025: 1 in 8 Adults Say They Are Currently Taking a GLP-1 Drug for Weight Loss, Diabetes, or Another Condition, Even as Half Say the Drugs Are Difficult to Afford," KFF, November 14, 2025; U.S. Census Bureau, "Annual Estimates of the Resident Population by Single Year of Age and Sex for the United States: April 1, 2020 to July 1, 2024," released June 2025.

Evidation estimates. The 7.79 million comes from net revenue divided by a constructed average price and composite adherence rate. But these limitations do not account for the difference and they do not change the directionality of the market gaps. The best explanation is that we do not know the actual size of the U.S. GLP-1 market because a large minority of it operates outside the branded supply chain.

THE COMPOUNDED GLP-1 MARKET

Compounding is the practice of combining, mixing, or altering drug ingredients to create a medication tailored to an individual patient's needs. There are two categories of compounding pharmacies in the United States:

1. 503A pharmacies that dispense individual prescriptions under state oversight

2. 503B outsourcing facilities that produce in bulk under federal manufacturing standards

Compounding does not include research-use-only peptides, counterfeit branded products, or drugs imported through cross-border online pharmacies.[59]

Compounding pharmacies are not required to report patient counts to the data aggregators that track branded prescriptions. The 503A pharmacies that fill individual compounded prescriptions are dispersed across thousands of facilities. The 503B outsourcing facilities that produce bulk GLP-1 powder by the kilogram operate under commercial agreements. Most compounded GLP-1s reach patients through direct-to-consumer digital health platforms that bypass standard pharmacy data capture, with most patients paying cash. Standard claims-based data infrastructure does not register any of this.

The size of the 2025 U.S. compounded GLP-1 market is a *wild guess*, according to Mark Mikhael, CEO of the 503B outsourcing facility Olympia Pharmaceuticals in Orlando, Florida. Mikhael told *KFF Health News* in mid-2024 that compounding pharmacies might account for up to 30% of the semaglutide sold in the United States.[60] Mikhael and other industry officials told the same outlet that several large compounding pharmacies were collectively supplying as many as 2 million American patients with semaglutide or tirzepatide.[61] Both numbers are industry self-estimates from compounders themselves. In May 2025, Goldman Sachs Research estimated that at least 1 million Americans were currently on compounded GLP-1. This was on the eve of the FDA's deadline for halting production of compounded semaglutide and tirzepatide.[62] We discuss this more in Chapter 5.

If Mikhael's upper estimate of 30% is right, approximately 9.7 million Americans were currently on a compounded GLP-1 in 2025, and 8 million of them were using it for weight loss. If the share is 20%, then that leaves 6.4 million Americans on compounded GLP-1s with 5.3 million of them for weight loss. If the share is 10%, that means 3.2 million Americans on compounded GLP-1s, with 2.7 million for weight loss (see Figure 2.7). The answer is somewhere between 1 and 10 million people. The compounded market could be larger than the branded market by this estimation, or merely one-eighth of it. A wild guess, indeed.

But we do know that people taking branded GLP-1s behave differently from those taking compounded GLP-1s. IQVIA is the healthcare data and analytics firm that aggregates U.S. prescription and claims data on behalf of the pharmaceutical industry and is widely treated as the industry standard for measuring branded drug utilization. IQVIA's GLP-1 data show a clear separation by the third month, with people on compounded GLP-1s discontinuing at meaningfully higher rates than people on branded GLP-1s (see Figures 2.8 and 2.9).

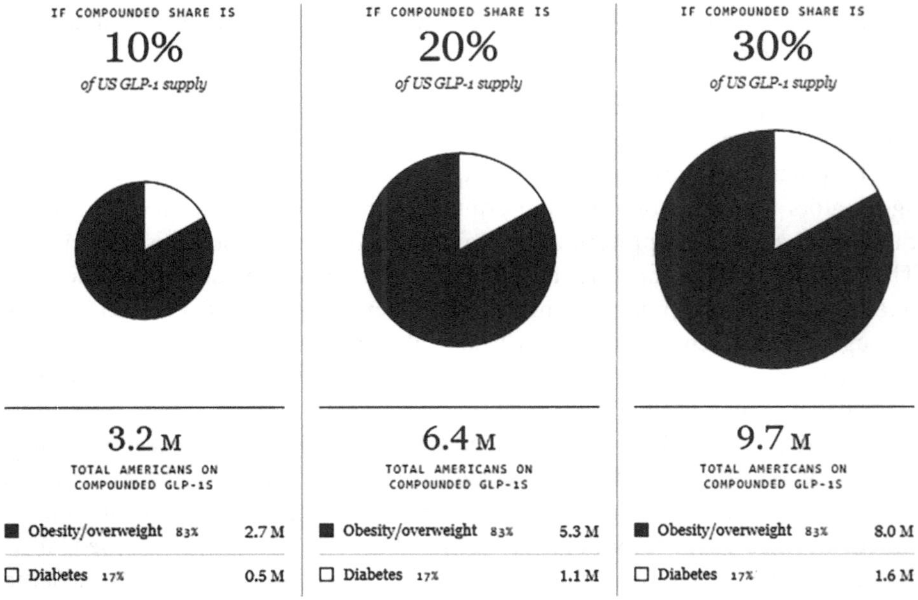

METHOD ***Each scenario applies an assumed compounded share to a 2025 US GLP-1 prescribed-user base of 32.2 million adults, then splits the resulting compounded population using the IQVIA-reported indication mix for tracked compounded volume (83 percent obesity/overweight, 17 percent diabetes). Circle area is proportional to total compounded users.***

Figure 2.7 Estimating the 2025 U.S. compounded GLP-1 market.

Sources: Luke Greenwalt et al., "Non-Traditional Channels: The Compounded GLP-1 Market," IQVIA Blog, October 22, 2025, https://www.iqvia.com/locations/united-states/blogs/2025/10/non-traditional-channels-the-compounded-glp-1-market; Kaiser Family Foundation, KFF Health Tracking Poll, October–November 2025; U.S. Census Bureau, 2025 adult population estimates. Author's calculation.

IQVIA attributes the gap to two factors: a subset of impulse buyers seeking rapid weight loss without long-term commitment, and the financial pressure of full out-of-pocket payment for compounded products without insurance coverage.[63] Switching from compounded to branded GLP-1s is rare, occurring in only 2% of patients each month. Once a patient is in the compounded channel, they tend to either continue compounded or drop off treatment entirely.

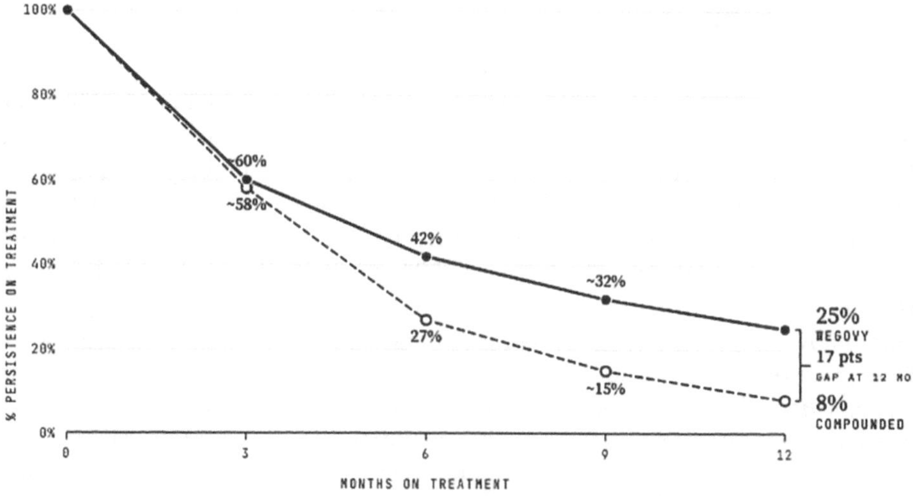

Figure 2.8 Persistence of patients on semaglutide for obesity. Figure reconstructed from *source*: Luke Greenwalt et al., "Non-Traditional Channels: The Compounded GLP-1 Market," IQVIA Blog, October 22, 2025, https://www.iqvia.com/locations/united-states/blogs/2025/10/non-traditional-channels-the-compounded-glp-1-market.

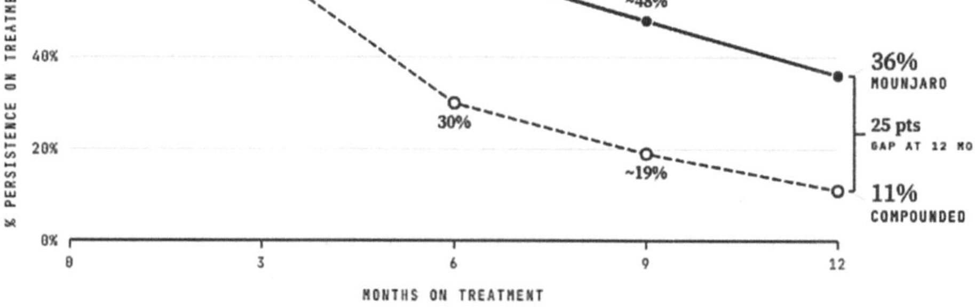

Figure 2.9 Persistence of patients on tirzepatide for obesity. Figure reconstructed from *source*: Luke Greenwalt et al., "Non-Traditional Channels: The Compounded GLP-1 Market," IQVIA Blog, October 22, 2025, https://www.iqvia.com/locations/united-states/blogs/2025/10/non-traditional-channels-the-compounded-glp-1-market.

The 55% Problem

The 15% market benchmark that health economists consider achievable for a modest expansion of access is far closer than revenue-first modeling suggests, but only if we count a massive parallel market of compounded medications that the FDA has said is illegal—a market that selects for patients who have a tendency to give up before their medication has time to produce sustained clinical benefit.

Under pressure from compounding markets, ATC for branded medications dropped by approximately 55% between 2024 and 2026. Branded market capture is expected to improve from 2% to just 7.2% in 2026. Branded price compression alone moves the needle by less than half the distance to the 15% benchmark. A 55% price reduction led to a five-percentage-point increase in branded market share. *This is the 55% Problem.* It is proof that two categories of market failure exist. The *cost and coverage* failure is being addressed through market forces and policy pressure. The *retention system* failure is in the infrastructure that surrounds the prescription. That is where most of the unrealized value sits, and it is the focus of this book.

The global context makes the retention system gap even more urgent. The World Obesity Federation projects that over 50% of the world's population will have a BMI over 25 by 2035.[64] Obesity rates continue to worsen in most countries. But in the United States, something different is happening. Rates are plateauing and may even be declining, with the strongest signal appearing in women over 40, precisely the demographic with the highest penetration of GLP-1 medications.[65]

This is a proof of concept for getting these medications to the right people and helping those people stay on them; it can shift the health of entire generations. Although, as drugmakers have discovered, this is easier said than done.

ENDNOTES

1. Keshob Sharma et al., *GLP-1 Coverage and Its Impact on Employment-Based Health Plan Premiums: A Simulation-Based Analysis* (Employee Benefit Research Institute, 2025); "Disease Overview: Understanding the Size and Scope of the U.S. Obesity Market," accessed December 21, 2025, https://www.iqvia.com/locations/united-states/blogs/2025/10/disease-overview-the-size-and-scope-of-the-us-obesity-market.
2. Brandon Aylward, "What's next for GLP-1 Innovation: A Primer on the Race Reshaping Pharma and Chronic Disease Care," Union, October 16, 2025, https://www.unionhealthcareinsight.com/post/glp-1-innovation-the-race-reshaping-pharma-and-chronic-disease-care.
3. Jennifer H. Hwang et al., "Lifetime Health Effects and Cost-Effectiveness of Tirzepatide and Semaglutide in U.S. Adults," *JAMA Health Forum* 6, no. 3 (2025): e245586, https://doi.org/10.1001/jamahealthforum.2024.5586.
4. Ibid.
5. Jardiance is empagliflozin, Farxiga is dapagliflozin, and Invokana is canagliflozin.
6. CDC, "National Diabetes Statistics Report," Diabetes, July 23, 2024, https://www.cdc.gov/diabetes/php/data-research/index.html; "Merck and Pfizer Launch Competitively Priced SGLT2 Inhibitor Steglatro for Type 2 Diabetes," MedPath, February 8, 2025, https://trial.medpath.com/news/0fb1a8b6d43ab97f/merck-and-pfizer-launch-competitively-priced-sglt2-inhibitor-steglatro-for-type-2-diabetes.
7. Author's calculation based on combined U.S. revenue: Jardiance ($4.3B), Farxiga ($1.75B), Invokana ($0.4–0.5B), and Steglatro ($0.1B). See Patricia Weiss, "Boehringer Ingelheim 2024 Sales up Forex-Adj 6.1%," Healthcare & Pharmaceuticals, *Reuters*, April 2, 2025, https://www.reuters.com/business/healthcare-pharmaceuticals/boehringer-ingelheim-2024-sales-up-forex-adj-61-2025-04-02/; *Eli Lilly and Company. Annual Report on Form 10-K (Year Ended December 31, 2024)*, Form 10-K (U.S. Securities and Exchange Commission, 2025).
8. Author's calculation. The CDC's National Diabetes Statistics Report (released January 21, 2026, using 2023 data) estimates 29.1 million Americans with diagnosed diabetes, and the CDC separately reports that type 2 diabetes accounts for approximately 90 to 95 percent of all diagnosed cases. Applying the lower end of that share yields approximately 26 million adults with diagnosed type 2 diabetes. See Centers for Disease Control and Prevention, "National Diabetes Statistics Report," last updated January 21, 2026, https://www.cdc.gov/diabetes/php/data-research/index.html; Centers for Disease Control and Prevention, "Type 2 Diabetes," last updated January 22, 2026, https://www.cdc.gov/diabetes/about/about-type-2-diabetes.html.

9. T. D. Müller et al., "Glucagon-like Peptide 1 (GLP-1)," *Molecular Metabolism* 30 (December 2019): 72–130, https://doi.org/10.1016/j.molmet.2019.09.010.
10. Emily J. Dhurandhar et al., "Food Noise: Definition, Measurement, and Future Research Directions," *Nutrition & Diabetes* 15 (2025): 30, https://doi.org/10.1038/s41387-025-00382-x.
11. Ralph A. DeFronzo and Muhammad Abdul-Ghani, "Sodium–Glucose Cotransporter 2 Inhibitors and the Kidney," *Diabetes Spectrum: A Publication of the American Diabetes Association* 34, no. 3 (2021): 225–34, https://doi.org/10.2337/ds20-0071.
12. Ania M. Jastreboff et al., "Tirzepatide Once Weekly for the Treatment of Obesity," *New England Journal of Medicine* 387, no. 3 (2022): 205–16, https://doi.org/10.1056/NEJMoa2206038.
13. Daniel J. Drucker, "Mechanisms of Action and Therapeutic Application of Glucagon-like Peptide-1," *Cell Metabolism* 27, no. 4 (2018): 740–56, https://doi.org/10.1016/j.cmet.2018.03.001; "FDA Approves First Medication for Obstructive Sleep Apnea," FDA News Release, FDA, December 27, 2024, https://www.fda.gov/news-events/press-announcements/fda-approves-first-medication-obstructive-sleep-apnea.
14. Atul Malhotra et al., "Tirzepatide for the Treatment of Obstructive Sleep Apnea and Obesity," *New England Journal of Medicine* 391, no. 13 (2024): 1193–205, https://doi.org/10.1056/NEJMoa2404881.
15. Arun J. Sanyal et al., "Phase 3 Trial of Semaglutide in Metabolic Dysfunction-Associated Steatohepatitis," *The New England Journal of Medicine* 392, no. 21 (2025): 2089–99, https://doi.org/10.1056/NEJMoa2413258.
16. "The Viral Side of Wellness: Lessons from GLP-1s," accessed December 22, 2025, https://www.mergeworld.com/insights/the-viral-side-of-wellness-lessons-from-glp1s.
17. Jakob Emerson, "Ozempic Is Becoming Cheaper," Healthcare News & Analysis, *Becker's Hospital Review*, December 2, 2024, https://www.beckershospitalreview.com/pharmacy/ozempic-is-becoming-cheaper/.
18. Graham Walker, "Mark Cuban: How I'd Reform Healthcare If I Were in Charge," How I Doctor (Offcall), April 3, 2025, https://www.offcall.com/learn/podcast/mark-cuban-interview-how-shark-tank-star-and-cost-plus-drugs-ceo-would-fix-healthcare.
19. Emerson, "Ozempic Is Becoming Cheaper"; Steven D. Pearson et al., "Affordable Access to GLP-1 Obesity Medications: Strategies to Guide Market Action and Policy Solutions in the U.S.," *Journal of Comparative Effectiveness Research* 14, no. 9 (2025): e250083, https://doi.org/10.57264/cer-2025-0083.
20. Ibid.
21. Grace A. Lin et al., *Semaglutide and Tirzepatide for Obesity: Effectiveness and Value* (Institute for Clinical and Economic Review, 2025).

22. "Obesity Deep Dive: How Payer Control Shaped the Market," IQVIA, 2025, https://www.iqvia.com/locations/united-states/blogs/2025/10/obesity-deep-dive-how-payer-control-shaped-the-market.
23. *Medicare Coverage of Anti-Obesity Medications*, ASPE Issue Brief (2024).
24. The White House, "Fact Sheet: President Donald J. Trump Announces Major Developments in Bringing Most-Favored-Nation Pricing to American Patients," The White House, November 6, 2025, https://www.whitehouse.gov/fact-sheets/2025/11/fact-sheet-president-donald-j-trump-announces-major-developments-in-bringing-most-favored-nation-pricing-to-american-patients/.
25. Lin et al., *Semaglutide and Tirzepatide for Obesity: Effectiveness and Value*.
26. Tom Murphy et al., "Trump Unveils Deal to Expand Coverage and Lower Costs on Obesity Drugs," *Magnolia Tribune*, November 6, 2025, https://magnoliatribune.com/2025/11/06/trump-unveils-deal-to-expand-coverage-and-lower-costs-on-obesity-drugs/.
27. Murphy et al., "Trump Unveils Deal to Expand Coverage and Lower Costs on Obesity Drugs"; "Eli Lilly (LLY) Q3 2025 Earnings Call Transcript," The Motley Fool, October 30, 2025, https://www.fool.com/earnings/call-transcripts/2025/10/30/eli-lilly-lly-q3-2025-earnings-call-transcript/.
28. Mina Kabiri et al., "The Societal Value of Broader Access to Anti-obesity Medications," *Obesity* 28, no. 2 (2020): 429–36, https://doi.org/10.1002/oby.22696.
29. Ibid.
30. Ibid.
31. Congressional Budget Office, *How Would Authorizing Medicare to Cover Anti-Obesity Medications Affect the Federal Budget?*, Publication 60441 (2024), https://www.cbo.gov/publication/60441; World Health Organ., "Obesity and Overweight."
32. This analysis excludes legacy anti-obesity medications (liraglutide, naltrexone/bupropion, phentermine/topiramate) for three reasons: clinical efficacy, commercial reality, and timing. Semaglutide and tirzepatide produce 13 to 20 percent weight loss; the older drugs produce 4 to 5 percent. Legacy drugs now represent under 5 percent of obesity medication revenue, and generics are arriving for both Saxenda and Qsymia.
33. Novo Nordisk A/S, *Financial Report for the Period 1 January 2024 to 31 December 2024*, Form 6-K (Washington, DC: U.S. Securities and Exchange Commission, February 5, 2025), https://www.sec.gov/Archives/edgar/data/353278/000162828025003924/caq42024.htm; Eli Lilly and Company, "Lilly Reports Full Q4 2024 Financial Results and Provides 2025 Guidance," news release, February 6, 2025, https://investor.lilly.com/news-releases/news-release-details/lilly-reports-full-q4-2024-financial-results-and-provides-2025.
34. Author's calculation. Off-label proportion derived from Kateri J. Spinelli et al., "Health Disparity Clusters of Off Label Prescriptions for Glucagon-Like Peptide 1 Receptor Agonists," *American Journal of Medicine Open* 13 (June 2025): 100100, https://doi.org/10.1016/j.ajmo.2025.100100, which found a median off-label rate

of 37.7 percent in a 2022 all-payer dataset of 3,688,430 prescriptions for type-2-diabetes-indicated GLP-1 RAs. Applied to 2024 U.S. Ozempic and Mounjaro net revenue derived from Novo Nordisk's Form 6-K (FY2024) and Eli Lilly's Q4 2024 earnings release.

35. Novo Nordisk A/S, *Financial Report for the Period 1 January 2025 to 31 December 2025*, Form 6-K (Washington, DC: U.S. Securities and Exchange Commission, February 4, 2026), https://www.sec.gov/Archives/edgar/data/0000353278/000035327826000006/caq42025.htm. Wegovy U.S. Operations sales of DKK 51,015 million converted to USD at the 2025 industry-conventional rate of approximately 6.8 DKK/USD.
36. Eli Lilly and Company, *Lilly Reports Fourth-Quarter 2025 Financial Results and Provides 2026 Guidance*, Form 8-K (Washington, DC: U.S. Securities and Exchange Commission, February 4, 2026), https://www.sec.gov/Archives/edgar/data/0000059478/000005947826000008/q425lillysalesandearningsp.htm. Worldwide Zepbound revenue of $13,542 million; tirzepatide is marketed for obesity as Zepbound in the United States, Canada, and Japan, with the United States representing the substantial majority of revenue.
37. Calculated from quarterly U.S. Mounjaro disclosures: Q1 2025 ($2,660 million), Q2 2025 ($3,300 million), Q3 2025 ($3,550 million), and Q4 2025 ($4,100 million). See Eli Lilly and Company, *Lilly Reports First-Quarter 2025 Financial Results and Highlights Pipeline Momentum*, Form 8-K (Washington, DC: U.S. Securities and Exchange Commission, May 1, 2025), https://www.sec.gov/Archives/edgar/data/0000059478/000005947825000129/q125lillysalesandearningsp.htm; Eli Lilly and Company, *Lilly Reports Second-Quarter 2025 Financial Results and Raises Guidance*, Form 8-K (Washington, DC: U.S. Securities and Exchange Commission, August 7, 2025), https://www.sec.gov/Archives/edgar/data/0000059478/000005947825000202/q225lillysalesandearningsp.htm; Eli Lilly and Company, *Lilly Reports Third-Quarter 2025 Financial Results, Highlights R&D Pipeline Momentum and Raises 2025 Guidance*, Form 8-K (Washington, DC: U.S. Securities and Exchange Commission, October 30, 2025), https://www.sec.gov/Archives/edgar/data/0000059478/000005947825000251/q325lillysalesandearningsp.htm; Eli Lilly and Company, *Lilly Reports Fourth-Quarter 2025 Financial Results and Provides 2026 Guidance*, Form 8-K (Washington, DC: U.S. Securities and Exchange Commission, February 4, 2026), https://www.sec.gov/Archives/edgar/data/0000059478/000005947826000008/q425lillysalesandearningsp.htm.
38. Novo Nordisk A/S, *Financial Report for the Period 1 January 2025 to 31 December 2025*, Form 6-K (Washington, DC: U.S. Securities and Exchange Commission, February 4, 2026), https://www.sec.gov/Archives/edgar/data/0000353278/000035327826000006/caq42025.htm. Novo Nordisk reports U.S. Operations GLP-1 diabetes care sales of DKK 97,771 million in 2025 without breaking out Ozempic and Rybelsus individually; U.S. Ozempic and Rybelsus values estimated from the U.S. GLP-1 diabetes care total after accounting for declining U.S. sales of Rybelsus and Victoza as disclosed in the same report.

39. Kevin J. Spinelli, Allison H. Oakes, Stella T. Chiu, Annie Sittler, John W. Sheets, and Sanjula Jain, "Health Disparity Clusters of Off Label Prescriptions for Glucagon-Like Peptide 1 Receptor Agonists," *American Journal of Medicine Open* 13 (June 2025): 100100, https://doi.org/10.1016/j.ajmo.2025.100100. Median county-level off-label prescribing rate of 37.7% (interquartile range 30.0%–46.3%) for GLP-1 receptor agonists approved for type 2 diabetes, applied to the off-label-eligible denominator (Ozempic, Mounjaro, Rybelsus); rounded to 38% for the calculation.
40. Don Tracy Editor Associate, "ICER Releases Cost Analysis Report on Obesity Treatments Semaglutide, Tirzepatide | Pharmaceutical Commerce," December 22, 2025, https://www.pharmaceuticalcommerce.com/view/icer-releases-cost-analysis-report-obesity-treatments-semaglutide-tirzepatide.
41. Zachary J. Ward et al., "Association of Body Mass Index with Health Care Expenditures in the United States by Age and Sex," *PloS One* 16, no. 3 (2021): e0247307, https://doi.org/10.1371/journal.pone.0247307.
42. Author's calculation based on estimated mean annual therapy cost derived from negotiated price ranges of $2,940–$4,200 for Wegovy and $2,940–$4,152 for Zepbound, yielding an average estimated annual cost of approximately $3,808 per patient. Oral formulations are held out of this scenario modeling because meaningful 2026 sales data do not yet exist.
43. Congressional Budget Office, *How Would Authorizing Medicare to Cover Anti-Obesity Medications Affect the Federal Budget?*; Pearson et al., "Affordable Access to GLP-1 Obesity Medications"; *Wegovy Market Size to Hit USD 24.53 Billion by 2034*, no. 6404 (Precedence Research, 2025), https://www.precedenceresearch.com/wegovy-market; House, "Fact Sheet"; Eli Lilly and Company, "Lilly Reports Third-Quarter 2025 Financial Results, Highlights R&D Pipeline Momentum and Raises 2025 Guidance"; Transcribing, "Novo Nordisk (NVO) Q3 2025 Earnings Transcript."
44. Ania M. Jastreboff et al., "Triple–Hormone-Receptor Agonist Retatrutide for Obesity—A Phase 2 Trial," *New England Journal of Medicine* 389, no. 6 (2023): 514–26, https://doi.org/10.1056/NEJMoa2301972.; W. Timothy Garvey et al., "Coadministered Cagrilintide and Semaglutide in Adults with Overweight or Obesity," *New England Journal of Medicine* 393, no. 7 (2025): 635–47, https://doi.org/10.1056/NEJMoa2502081.
45. FDA, "FDA Approves First Medication for Obstructive Sleep Apnea."
46. Adam J. Fein, "The Gross-to-Net Bubble Hits $356 Billion in 2024," Twitter, Drug Channels, December 12, 2025, https://x.com/DrugChannels/status/1999468084650725850.
47. The Truveris Team, "4 Key Stages of the PBM Contract Lifecycle," *Truveris*, 2025, https://truveris.com/pbm-contract-lifecycle/.
48. Steven D. Pearson et al., "Affordable Access to GLP-1 Obesity Medications: Strategies to Guide Market Action and Policy Solutions in the U.S.," *Journal of Comparative Effectiveness Research* 14, no. 9 (2025): e250083, https://doi.org/10.57264/cer-2025-0083.

49. Alex Montero, Grace Sparks, Marley Presiado, and Liz Hamel, "KFF Health Tracking Poll May 2024: The Public's Use and Views of GLP-1 Drugs," KFF, May 10, 2024, https://www.kff.org/health-costs/poll-finding/kff-health-tracking-poll-may-2024-the-publics-use-and-views-of-glp-1-drugs/.
50. Robert Bozick, Shannon D. Donofry, and Katherine M. Rancaño, *New Weight Loss Drugs: GLP-1 Agonist Use and Side Effects in the United States* (Santa Monica, CA: RAND Corporation, 2025), https://www.rand.org/pubs/research_reports/RRA4153-1.html.
51. "Behaviors and Characteristics of Current and Previous Users of Glucagon-Like Peptide-1 Receptor Agonists (GLP-1) in an Online Health Community" (abstract EPH32, presented at the International Society for Pharmacoeconomics and Outcomes Research Annual Meeting, Atlanta, GA, May 5–8, 2024), referenced in Evidation, "Evidation Shares Real-World Data on GLP-1 Use and Social Determinants of Health at ISPOR 2024," May 6, 2024, https://www.businesswire.com/news/home/20240506471832/en/Evidation-Shares-Real-World-Data-on-GLP-1-Use-and-Social-Determinants-of-Health-at-ISPOR-2024.
52. Ashley Kirzinger et al., "KFF Health Tracking Poll November 2025: 1 in 8 Adults Say They Are Currently Taking a GLP-1 Drug for Weight Loss, Diabetes, or Another Condition, Even As Half Say the Drugs Are Difficult to Afford," KFF, November 14, 2025, https://www.kff.org/public-opinion/poll-1-in-8-adults-say-they-are-currently-taking-a-glp-1-drug-for-weight-loss-diabetes-or-another-condition-even-as-half-say-the-drugs-are-difficult-to-afford/.
53. House, "Fact Sheet"; Brian Buntz, "Novo Cuts GLP-1 Prices 70%, but Semaglutide Revenue Could Grow in 2026," *Drug Discovery and Development*, November 17, 2025, https://www.drugdiscoverytrends.com/novo-slashes-us-glp-1-prices-by-up-to-70-but-2026-semaglutide-revenue-could-hold-steady-or-even-grow/.
54. U.S. Census Bureau, "Annual Estimates of the Resident Population by Single Year of Age and Sex for the United States: April 1, 2020 to July 1, 2024," released June 2025, https://www.census.gov/data/tables/time-series/demo/popest/2020s-national-detail.html.
55. Alex Montero, Grace Sparks, Marley Presiado, and Liz Hamel, "KFF Health Tracking Poll May 2024: The Public's Use and Views of GLP-1 Drugs," KFF, May 10, 2024, https://www.kff.org/health-costs/poll-finding/kff-health-tracking-poll-may-2024-the-publics-use-and-views-of-glp-1-drugs/.
56. Centers for Disease Control and Prevention, "National Diabetes Statistics Report," last updated January 21, 2026, https://www.cdc.gov/diabetes/php/data-research/index.html.
57. Yunwen Xu, Justin B. Echouffo Tcheugui, Josef Coresh, Morgan E. Grams, Elizabeth Selvin, Michael Fang, and Jung-Im Shin. "Trends in Obesity and Glucagon-like Peptide-1 Receptor Agonist Prescriptions in Type 1 Diabetes in the United States." *Diabetes, Obesity and Metabolism* 27, no. 6 (June 2025): 2967–2976. https://doi.org/10.1111/dom.16300.

58. D. Do, T. Lee, S. K. Peasah, C. B. Good, A. Inneh, and U. Patel. GLP-1 Receptor Agonist Discontinuation Among Patients With Obesity and/or Type 2 Diabetes. *JAMA Network Open*. 2024 May 1;7(5):e2413172. doi:10.1001/jamanetworkopen.2024.13172. PMID: 38787563; PMCID: PMC11127113. PDC of 54.4 percent at twelve months reported among the obesity-only cohort.
59. U.S. Food and Drug Administration, "Human Drug Compounding," accessed May 19, 2026, https://www.fda.gov/drugs/guidance-compliance-regulatory-information/human-drug-compounding; U.S. Food and Drug Administration, "Compounding and the FDA: Questions and Answers," accessed May 19, 2026, https://www.fda.gov/drugs/human-drug-compounding/compounding-and-fda-questions-and-answers; U.S. Food and Drug Administration, "Drug Compounding and Drug Shortages," accessed May 19, 2026, https://www.fda.gov/drugs/human-drug-compounding/drug-compounding-and-drug-shortages.
60. Arthur Allen, "Why Millions Are Trying FDA-Authorized Alternatives to Big Pharma's Weight Loss Drugs," *KFF Health News*, July 23, 2024, https://kffhealthnews.org/health-industry/glp1-compounding-pharmacies-wegovy-zepbound-copycat-drugs-shortages/.
61. Ibid.
62. Goldman Sachs Research, "The Anti-Obesity Drug Market May Prove Smaller Than Expected," May 22, 2025, https://www.goldmansachs.com/insights/articles/the-anti-obesity-drug-market-may-prove-smaller-than-expected.
63. Luke Greenwalt, Jeff Thiesen, Teddy Landsman, Anika LaFazia, and Mitchell Haynes, "Non-Traditional Channels: The Compounded GLP-1 Market," IQVIA Blog, October 22, 2025, https://www.iqvia.com/locations/united-states/blogs/2025/10/non-traditional-channels-the-compounded-glp-1-market.
64. *World Obesity Atlas 2025* (World Obesity Federation, 2025).
65. Benjamin Rader, Rotem Hazan, and John S. Brownstein, "Changes in Adult Obesity Trends in the U.S.," *JAMA Health Forum* 5, no. 12 (2024): e243685, https://doi.org/10.1001/jamahealthforum.2024.3685.

CHAPTER 3

WHY YOU ARE READING, AND I AM WRITING THIS BOOK

Wayne is sitting in his home office on a Thursday afternoon. He's 64 years old and six feet eight inches tall. Even seated at his desk, his head rises above the double monitors. His phone is on speaker. His doctor's voice comes through: "I don't know what else to try. Maybe just stop it."

"Okay," Wayne says. "I think that's what I'll do."

Wayne is self-employed, runs a small business, and pays out of pocket for everything. When his family doctor started him on Ozempic before the weight-loss hype, it was to handle his prediabetes and metabolic risk. He's been on Ozempic for eight months, paying out of pocket. He's lost 15 pounds, bringing his weight down from his highest of 350 pounds. His fasting glucose has dropped. But every time he tries to increase beyond 0.25 mg, the same pattern plays out.

- Week 1: Wayne starts taking 0.25 mg. He is optimistic. His appetite is noticeably reduced. He feels like this might actually work.
- Week 3: He's missed two doses in a row. Not intentionally, just forgot. He takes another 0.25mg 18 days after the first.
- Week 4: His doctor's protocol calls for increasing to 0.5 mg. He's not sure if he should, given the missed doses, but the printed instructions say to increase after week 4. He takes the higher dose. Within hours, the nausea hits. Not mild queasiness but full-body misery. The symptoms last three days and prevent him from seeing clients and earning a living.

He stops semaglutide entirely. Waits two weeks. Tries again at 0.25 mg. The same pattern plays out. A good start, missed doses, confusion about timing, another escalation attempt, followed by another crash.

This cycle repeated three times over eight months. Each time, the gap between doses got longer. Each restart felt more demoralizing. Each crash reinforced that this medication *doesn't work for him*. Wayne makes a rational decision. He stops spending significant money on something that makes him feel terrible when he tries to increase his dose.

Wayne was a high school football star, the kind of athlete who filled a doorway. He focused on martial arts through his twenties and thirties. Being an athlete isn't something you do; it's something you are. He still carries that, the way he moves, his presence.

But his appetite and portion sizes were programmed during years of rapid growth and enormous energy expenditure. That pattern proved difficult to change when the intense training stopped. His body mass index (BMI) climbed from 28 kg/m^2 in his teens to 38 kg/m^2 in his forties, and to nearly 50 kg/m^2 in his fifties. BMI is an imperfect proxy for health, particularly at extremes of height and muscularity. It cannot distinguish between fat and muscle, doesn't account for where weight is carried, and was never designed to assess individual health. But Wayne's trajectory told a story BMI alone couldn't. His weight gain was mostly in his abdomen—the pattern most strongly correlated with cardiovascular and metabolic risk.

The diagnoses accumulated. He was diagnosed with elevated cholesterol in his fifties, then hypertension, then prediabetes, and most recently atrial fibrillation, which is an irregular heart rate that increases his lifetime risk of stroke and heart failure. He's on five medications now, plus semaglutide. The regimen includes a beta-blocker, an ACE inhibitor, metformin, a statin, and an anticoagulant.

Before he started semaglutide, he got extremely sleepy after meals, an energy drop that affected his work performance and mood. A couple of hours later, the hunger would come back, urgently.

Wayne was diagnosed with attention deficit hyperactivity disorder (ADHD) late in life. Stimulant medications and behavioral support earlier in his life might have helped with the appetite dysregulation common to the condition. But now the atrial fibrillation makes stimulants contraindicated. The treatment that might have helped him most is much riskier because of a condition related to his weight. He might have avoided that condition if he'd had the ADHD diagnosis and treatment decades earlier.

This is the tangle of obesity and metabolic health in a real person's life. Wayne faces two possible futures with and without sustained treatment for obesity.

In version one, his A1c, the standard measure of glucose control, drops from 6.2% to 5.7% and stays there. The 15-pound loss he's achieved becomes 60 pounds over 18 months. His LDL cholesterol falls below the danger zone. At 72, he is still sparring at the dojo. At 78, he is still driving, cooking, and living independently.

In version two, his A1c drifts upward from 6.5% to 6.8% and then to 7.1%. Prediabetes becomes diabetes. He is even more short of breath at rest. His cardiologist diagnoses him with early heart failure, and his medication cocktail goes from six to nine daily medications overnight. He adds a diuretic, an SGLT2 inhibitor, and a second blood pressure medication. At 70, he's struggling with a complex medication regimen. At 73, he has his first hospitalization for acute decompensated heart failure. At 76, he contemplates whether he can continue living independently.

I wish this were hyperbole. It is kind of banal if you have ever worked in a North American hospital. More than one *Wayne* is in every emergency room on the continent as you read this.

I am writing this book because I want the first version to become the norm.

I'm a physician managing chronic disease. My scope is patients who need treatment to help them access medication, stay on it, and achieve outcomes that change their disease trajectory.

The cultural conversation about these medications is broader. They're being prescribed to people who don't need them—and that's a real problem.[1] I carry no brief for our culture's obsession with thinness. But that conversation belongs elsewhere. This book is about the gap between the patients who need treatment and the system that fails to deliver it.

That's my stake in this. Now let me tell you yours.

You're reading this book because you're trying to make sense of the obesity economy, and something about it does not add up. Noom closed its Series F at a $3.7 billion post-money valuation in May 2021. By late 2024, secondary-market trading valued the company at approximately $1 billion, a 73% decline.[2] Ro and Hims & Hers face approximately 50% annual customer churn (the rate at which subscribers cancel and stop paying), and cross-selling across conditions is lower than projected.[3]

These companies optimized for acquisition: how many customers could they sign up and at what price? They spent whatever they had to spend to grow. They did not build what was needed to retain customers.

Business strategists call this the difference between market share and wallet share. Market share is how many people buy from you. Wallet share is how much each customer keeps buying from you over time.[4] You can buy market share with pricing and advertising. Wallet share has to be earned, month after month, through lasting value that keeps the customer coming back.[5] By increasing customer retention rates, companies can often achieve higher profits than by acquiring new customers, as existing customers are more likely to buy again and spend more.[6]

In chronic disease, wallet share depends on the patient staying well and feeling like your solution is part of that. A patient who quits a GLP-1 at month four leaves behind the cost of acquiring it and none of the revenue. A patient who continues treatment for three years generates five to seven times the revenue of one who churns at 12 months.

The digital health companies that grew fastest during the 2021 to 2023 boom are now confronting this transition. Hims & Hers, Ro, and their competitors built extraordinary customer acquisition machines. They are now pivoting toward retention infrastructure. This includes coaching programs, personalization, and wraparound services that keep patients engaged beyond the first prescription. Some will succeed. Many will not. The winners will be those who recognize that wallet share in obesity medicine requires far more than a prescription.

This is the commercial translation of what I see in the exam room. Patient success and customer lifetime value are the same thing, measured differently. In obesity treatment, the right intervention at the right time determines whether a patient continues or quits. This includes a coaching check-in that explains why the on-off pattern of medication causes exactly those symptoms and guidance on how and when to restart properly. These interventions prevent discontinuation, thereby preserving revenue. The question is *how* to deliver them—not as expensive custom care, not as generic commodity access, but as something scalable that actually works. We can probably agree that the answer lives somewhere between commodity and perfectly customized care.

Supply chain management has a framework called the *7Rs*, which covers the right *product*, right *quantity*, right *condition*, right *place*, right *time*, right *customer*, and right *price*. A grocery store that carries the right bread at the right price is still in a difficult situation if the bread is stale, or the store is 30 miles away, or the door is locked when the customer gets off work. Miss one *R* and the system fails the customer.[7] In obesity medicine, the *right price* is finally getting close—the other six *Rs* are not.

I help patients like Wayne through the tricky parts of their care every week in my practice. I know that success is possible when support exists. All of it is doable at scale without requiring direct handholding from a physician. The companies that build this infrastructure will capture wallet share. The companies that do not will find themselves competing on price alone, watching patients churn at rates that make the business unsustainable.

WHERE YOU ARE SITTING

You are probably reading this from one of three seats—the pharmaceutical strategy seat, the product-building seat, or the investor's seat—and from each seat, the picture looks the same.

From a *pharmaceutical strategy seat*, two sets of numbers refuse to reconcile. Eli Lilly and Novo Nordisk have each announced billions in new manufacturing capacity.[8] Only 15% of patients remain on therapy after two years.[9] Goldman Sachs is forecasting a structural shift from *price-for-margin* to *price-for-volume*.[10]

Government negotiations are pushing Medicare prices way down. But how will you keep the patients that lower prices will attract?

From a *product-building seat*, Hims & Hers has become one of the largest prescribers of compounded weight-loss medications in the United States. Their chief product officer, Dheerja Kaur, describes the opportunity as moving *upper funnel*, beyond dispensing medication toward diagnostics, personalization, and holistic health management.[11] But the prescription is only the start of the problem. Patients without type 2 diabetes discontinue at 64.8% within a year.[12] Something about the diabetes population's existing care infrastructure and diabetes itself produces better retention. Blue Health Intelligence has shown where the leverage points sit. Each additional provider visit increases the likelihood that a patient reaches the 12-week persistence milestone by roughly 60%, and patients cared for by obesity medicine specialists are 22% more likely to persist than those cared for by primary care physicians. Specialists write fewer than 10% of total prescriptions.[13] There is a delivery model that works, but it cannot scale.

From an *investor's seat*, the patent cliff is already visible. Semaglutide's main U.S. patent expires in December 2031; tirzepatide's patent expires in 2036.[14] Canada—where I practice—is providing a preview. Generic semaglutide is entering the 2026 market, and companies like Hims & Hers have acquired Canadian assets to position for a higher-volume, lower-margin future.[15] Chapter 2 showed that even a 55% price reduction moved projected 2026 U.S. branded market capture from 2% to about 7.2%, still barely half of what health economists consider achievable.[16] We can't resolve the public health crisis of obesity on the back of compounders because, by nature, their business objectives are not aligned with the clinical ones.

WHAT THIS BOOK IS FOR

This book is about helping people who want treatment gain access to it and stay on it. For the first time, we have pharmacological tools that help people eat fewer calories than they burn, comfortably, without the enormous effort and distress that characterize dieting. GLP-1 medications are imperfect, but they represent a vast improvement over the hunger rages and metabolic whiplash that people experience when they try to restrict calories through willpower alone.

WHY THIS MARKET IS COUNTERINTUITIVE

Obesity medicine confounds people. The market operates by rules that run counter to intuition in other therapeutic categories.

Invisible Success

Weight loss itself is visible. Chapter 2 discussed the physical changes that drive social proof and market demand. But many of the most meaningful clinical outcomes remain invisible to everyone except the patients and their care teams.

When someone weighs 300 pounds and then loses 15% of their body weight, they weigh 255 pounds. They are still in a large body. To an outside observer, they may not look thin, but this could be a medical mission accomplished. Their A1c has most likely normalized, their blood pressure medications have been reduced, and their joint pain has improved enough that they can walk up stairs easily.

The metabolic reprieve is invisible, as are reductions in cardiovascular risk and improvement in sleep apnea severity. When a patient tells me the *food noise*—that constant mental preoccupation with eating—has quieted for the first time in years, I cannot prove that to an insurer. No lab value captures the relief of a brain that has finally stopped screaming about food. This invisibility creates a measurement problem. The outcomes that matter most to long-term health do not photograph well and do not show up on a scale in ways that feel proportionate to the effort required.

The Paradox of Discontinuation

Patients sometimes quit because the treatment worked. This is what researchers call paradoxical discontinuation, when patients stop therapy because it succeeded.[17] A patient reaches their goal weight, feels transformed, and decides the medication was temporary scaffolding rather than ongoing treatment for a chronic disease. Then the weight returns.

The STEP 1 trial extension showed that patients regained two-thirds of the weight they had lost within a year of stopping semaglutide.[18] The biology reasserts itself. The body defends its previous set point. Without the medication, the appetite signals return to their previous intensity.

This pattern is particularly common in patients without other metabolic diagnoses. Someone treating obesity alone is more likely to view the medication as a temporary intervention than someone managing both obesity and type 2 diabetes, which has a clearer framework for chronic disease management.

The Participation Problem

Statins lower cholesterol regardless of whether the patient thinks about them. Obesity medications require participation. The medication changes appetite signals, but the patient still has to learn new eating patterns, manage side effects, adjust protein intake, and navigate social situations where food is central.

WHAT CLINICAL TRIALS ACTUALLY PROVIDE

Clinical trials are designed to eliminate noise so researchers can detect signals. When testing whether a molecule works, you need to isolate its effect from confounding variables. This requires controlling the environment in ways that do not translate to routine care.

Dave Ricks, CEO of Eli Lilly, described this in a 2025 interview with Stripe's founders. The median clinical trial enrollee costs approximately $40,000 because sponsors essentially run a *premium healthcare system for participants.*[19] Medications are provided at no cost. Monitoring is frequent, and clinical support is intensive. Side effects are managed proactively. Every barrier that might cause a patient to quit in the real world is systematically removed so the trial can answer two narrow scientific questions: (1) Does this drug do what we think it does? and (2) Is this drug safe for human use?

The big downward moves in price by Novo Nordisk and Eli Lilly are important, but they are not enough. In Phase 3 clinical trials, where costs are eliminated, clinical support is intensive, and monitoring is frequent, retention rates approach 90%. In the SURMOUNT-1 trial, approximately 90% of participants completed the 72-week treatment period.[20] This represents the upper bound of what is possible when the system is optimized for patient success.

THE RETENTION PROBLEM

In real-world settings, retention collapses. A large study of 125,474 adults in the United States found that among patients with obesity and no diabetes, the one-year discontinuation rate was 64.8%, meaning only 35.2% remained on therapy.[21] Wayne is one of those 125,474 adults, statistically speaking. By year two, only about 15.6% of those who started GLP-1 therapy for weight loss remained on treatment.[22]

Blue Health Intelligence has one of the most comprehensive commercial health care databases in the United States. Their 2024 report on real-world retention regarding GLP-1 treatment showed that 30% of commercially insured patients discontinue within the first month. By week 12, when clinical guidelines suggest meaningful weight loss begins, 58% have already stopped treatment.[23]

Patients face out-of-pocket costs, supply chain disruptions, misinformation, and side effects without proactive management. The 50-point retention gap between clinical trials and the real world is a measure of everything the real-world system fails to provide.[24]

The Growth Ceiling

The current *very high* treatment-discontinuation rate is not merely expensive; it creates an absolute ceiling on how large any company can grow, regardless of how much money it spends on marketing.

Every subscription business, whether it sells streaming video or chronic disease management, operates under the same constraint. The maximum number of customers you can ever maintain equals your monthly new customer additions divided by your monthly churn rate.[25] A company that adds 10,000 new patients each month and loses 8% of its existing patients each month will see its patient base climb steadily and then flatten near 125,000. Doubling the new patient additions to 20,000 per month raises the ceiling to 250,000. Cutting churn in half, from 8% to 4%, reaches the same 250,000 ceiling on half the marketing spend. The churn rate, not the marketing budget, determines how big any company can ever become (see Figure 3.1).

Most subscription health companies frame retention in terms of customer acquisition cost (CAC) payback, with high performers recovering CAC in five to seven months and the rest of the field targeting 12 months. Payback windows indicate whether a company can afford to acquire the next patient. They cannot predict where the company's ceiling will sit. For that, you need to know what fraction of patients will be leaving each month.[26] The focus on acquisition cost recovery is too narrow to capture the threat of poor retention to overall growth.

To understand why, think about filling a bathtub that has a leaky drain. A small leak is manageable. Turn the faucet a little higher, and the water rises. But the bigger the leak gets, the harder the faucet has to work. At some point, the leak is so large that water escapes as fast as it comes in. The tub never fills, no matter how wide you open the tap. You need to fix the drain in order to keep the tub filled.

Digital health platforms for obesity are running their faucets at full blast. Hims & Hers spent $283 million on marketing in a single quarter of 2024.[27] Unfortunately, these companies are filling bathtubs with gaping holes in the bottom. They can grow quickly at first, when their patient bases are small and the absolute churn rate is manageable. But as they scale, churn scales with them, until new additions merely replace departures and growth stops entirely.

This is not a hypothetical concern for the future. It explains why the obesity medicine market is underperforming despite billions in marketing investment, despite genuine demand, and despite medications that work. Chapter 2 traced how the U.S. market moved from under 2% capture in 2024 to a projected 7.2% in 2026, with the 15% benchmark achievable only if compounded medications are counted. The market's apparent climb runs through an infrastructure that accounts for churn (patients who pay out of pocket and leave within months) and assumes they

Patient base over 60 months. Each scenario starts from zero patients and follows $P(t+1) = (1 - churn) \times P(t) + additions$.

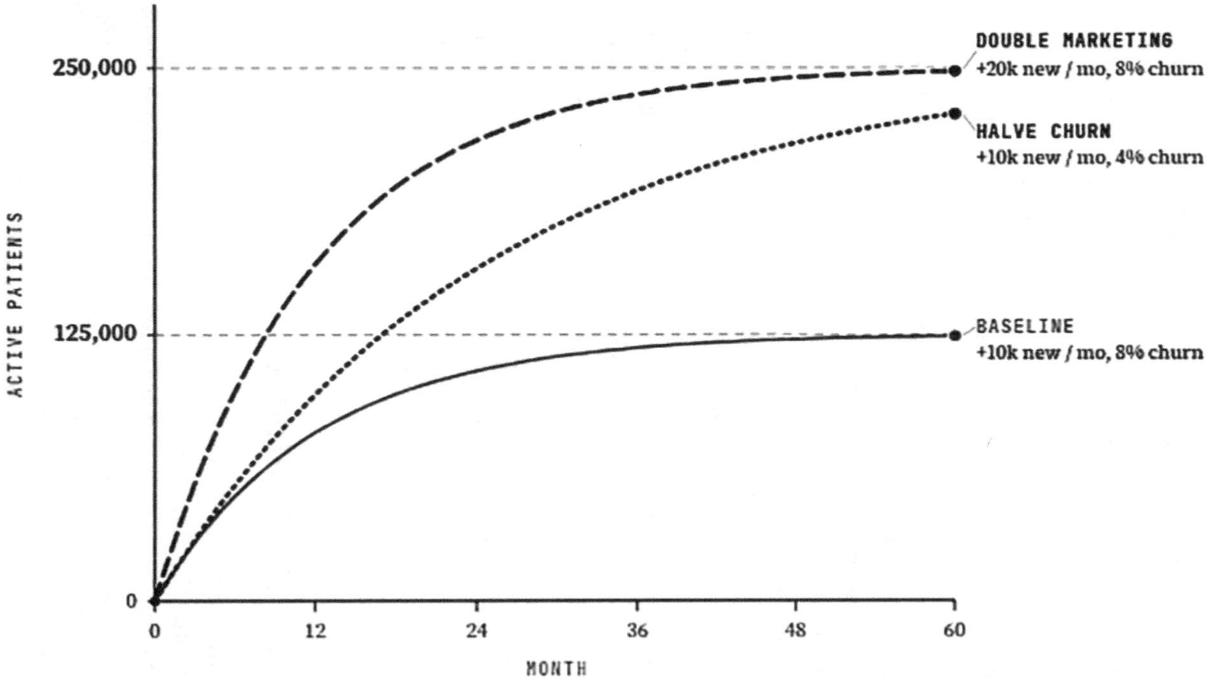

Dashed reference lines mark the ceiling each scenario approaches (monthly additions ÷ monthly churn rate). The halve-churn curve is still climbing at month 60 — retention reaches the same ceiling by a slower, more durable path.

Figure 3.1 The growth ceiling is set by churn, not by marketing spend.

will be replaced by the next cohort facing the same barriers. Both branded and compounded channels are pouring water into bathtubs with the drains wide open.

At this stage, fixing the drain matters more than opening the faucet wider. A company with modest marketing but 80% annual retention will eventually surpass a company with aggressive marketing but 50% retention, because the first company's ceiling is twice as high.

TWO CATEGORIES OF SOLVABLE PROBLEMS

Chapter 2 demonstrated that even dramatic price compression does not close the gap between actual market capture and what health economists consider achievable. The retention data helps explain this.

When researchers examine why patients discontinue treatment, the attribution splits roughly in half. Approximately half cite non-cost factors such as side effects, perceived lack of necessity, and supply shortages, while the other half cite cost and coverage.[28] This revisits the two categories of solvable problems described in Chapter 2: (1) cost and coverage and (2) the retention system. The cost-and-coverage problem is being addressed. List prices are falling. Medicare is negotiating. Direct-to-consumer channels are emerging. Wayne's story shows how cost barriers create impossible trade-offs, but market forces and policy pressure are working on this problem.

The retention system is where the unrealized value sits. This is 44% to 70% of discontinuation driven by factors other than cost. Part II examines how other companies have handled the gap between acquiring customers and retaining them: Apple's pricing correction, Ticketmaster's scarcity trap, Peloton's retention collapse, and Zara's responsive supply chain.

HOW VALUE GETS CAPTURED

Most markets involve a real tension between helping people and making money. In obesity medicine, the tension is mostly gone if the former is done well. The interventions that improve patient outcomes are the same ones that improve commercial outcomes. Expanding access serves both equity and market expansion. Keeping patients healthy serves both clinical obligation and retention economics.

The companies that see this will build accordingly. The companies that keep treating patients as transactions, optimizing for acquisition while ignoring the 65% who walk out the door, will become case studies in missed opportunities.

WHAT THIS BOOK OFFERS

- **Part I** establishes the gap. It shows the market mathematics and introduces you to Sarah and Wayne. It explains why 15% U.S. penetration by 2030 is the table stakes—the floor the industry should already be clearing. The 2026-and-beyond project is not about acquiring patients faster; it is about helping patients succeed on their own terms.
- **Part II** examines how other companies have faced the gap between acquiring customers and retaining them—some successfully, some catastrophically. Apple learned to build infrastructure before dropping prices. Ticketmaster created artificial scarcity that bred resentment and competitors. Peloton achieved stunning retention, only to lose it. Zara built a supply chain that responds to what customers actually want. These are case studies in what happens when companies confront the same choices now facing those in obesity medicine. Build for retention, or optimize for acquisition and watch value evaporate.
- **Part III** presents two things. The first thing is the infrastructure required to raise the ceiling in obesity medicine is shared and organized around seven components that together drive patient success from the first prescription through lasting transformation. The second thing is a measurement framework to determine whether the infrastructure is working, with metrics that track what patients do, what programs build, and what clinical outcomes may ensue. We return to the experiences with Sarah and Wayne to show what each component would have provided for them, and what the measurements would have revealed.

THE INVITATION

When I invite business leaders to think beyond acquisition, most stop listening. I'm asking you to keep an open mind about how value emerges from this space in 2026 and beyond. The way forward runs through patient success, which means investing in patients. We are all learning what this looks like for the future of medicine and our society itself.

ENDNOTES

1. Hassan E. Muhammad and Asad Ali Ahmed Cheema, "From Prescription to Trend: The Misuse of Ozempic in the Age of Social Media," *Annals of Medicine and Surgery* 87, no. 10 (2025): 6876–77, https://doi.org/10.1097/MS9.0000000000003801.
2. "Noom Announces $540 Million in Growth Funding to Further Accelerate Expansion of Its Digital Health Platform," *Silver Lake*, May 25, 2021, https://www.silverlake.com/noom-announces-540-million-in-growth-funding-to-further-accelerate-expansion-of-its-digital-health-platform/; Jan-Erik Asplun and Marcelo Ballve, *Noom*, Equity Research (Sacra, 2025), https://sacra.com/c/noom/.
3. Rohit Kaul, "Ro and the Telehealth Capital Cycle," Sacra, October 6, 2022, https://sacra.com/research/ro-telehealth-capital-cycle/.
4. Timothy L. Keiningham, Lerzan Aksoy, Alexander Buoye, and Bruce Cooil, "Customer Loyalty Isn't Enough. Grow Your Share of Wallet," *Harvard Business Review* 89, no. 10 (October 2011): 29–31.
5. Timothy L. Keiningham, Lerzan Aksoy, Luke Williams, and Alexander J. Buoye, *The Wallet Allocation Rule: Winning the Battle for Share* (Hoboken, NJ: John Wiley & Sons, 2015).
6. Frederick F. Reichheld with Thomas Teal, *The Loyalty Effect: The Hidden Force Behind Growth, Profits, and Lasting Value* (Boston: Harvard Business School Press, 1996), 36.
7. John Coyle and Ed, *The Management of Business Logistics: A Supply Chain Perspective*, 7th ed. (2003).
8. Eli Lilly and Company, "Lilly Reports Third-Quarter 2025 Financial Results, Highlights R&D Pipeline Momentum and Raises 2025 Guidance," October 25, 2025, https://www.prnewswire.com/news-releases/lilly-reports-third-quarter-2025-financial-results-highlights-rd-pipeline-momentum-and-raises-2025-guidance-302599148.html.
9. Prime Therapeutics, "Prime Continues to Lead Industry on GLP-1 Research: 1 in 7 Stays on GLP-1 Drugs for Weight Loss after Two Years," July 10, 2024, https://www.primetherapeutics.com/w/prime-continues-to-lead-industry-on-glp-1-research-1-in-7-stays-on-glp-1-drugs-for-weight-loss-after-two-years.
10. Goldman Sachs, "The Anti-Obesity Drug Market May Prove Smaller than Expected," Goldman Sachs Insights, May 22, 2025, https://www.goldmansachs.com/insights/articles/the-anti-obesity-drug-market-may-prove-smaller-than-expected; The White House, "Fact Sheet: President Donald J. Trump Announces Major Developments in Bringing Most-Favored-Nation Pricing to American Patients," The White House, November 6, 2025, https://www.whitehouse.gov/fact-sheets/2025/11/fact-sheet-president-donald-j-trump-announces-major-developments-in-bringing-most-favored-nation-pricing-to-american-patients/.

11. *Hims & Hers CPO on Building Delightful Products in Regulated Markets*, directed by Product School, 2025, 42:00, https://www.youtube.com/watch?v=8ELnsaC7YZg.
12. Patricia J. Rodriguez et al., "Discontinuation and Reinitiation of Dual-Labeled GLP-1 Receptor Agonists Among U.S. Adults With Overweight or Obesity," *JAMA Network Open* 8, no. 1 (2025): e2457349, https://doi.org/10.1001/jamanetworkopen.2024.57349.
13. Blue Health Intelligence, *Real-World Trends in GLP-1 Treatment Persistence and Prescribing for Weight Management* (Blue Health Intelligence, 2024).
14. Novo Nordisk, "Product Patents," Novo Nordisk USA, accessed April 28, 2026, https://www.novonordisk-us.com/content/nncorp/us/en_us/products/product-patents.html; U.S. Food and Drug Administration, *Approved Drug Products with Therapeutic Equivalence Evaluations (Orange Book)*, patent entry for U.S. Patent No. 8,129,343 (semaglutide), expiration December 5, 2031, https://www.accessdata.fda.gov/scripts/cder/ob/.
15. Chris Hannay, "Hims & Hers Acquires Livewell in Canada in Anticipation of Generic Ozempic," *The Globe and Mail*, January 5, 2025, https://www.theglobeandmail.com/business/economy/article-hims-hers-launches-in-canada-in-anticipation-of-generic-ozempic/.
16. Author's calculation based on Chapter 2 scenario modeling.
17. Rodriguez et al., "Discontinuation and Reinitiation of Dual-Labeled GLP-1 Receptor Agonists Among U.S. Adults With Overweight or Obesity."
18. John P. H. Wilding et al., "Weight Regain and Cardiometabolic Effects after Withdrawal of Semaglutide: The STEP 1 Trial Extension," *Diabetes, Obesity & Metabolism* 24, no. 8 (2022): 1553–64, https://doi.org/10.1111/dom.14725.
19. *Dave Ricks, CEO of Eli Lilly, on GLP-1s and the Business of Pharma*, directed by Stripe, 2025, https://www.youtube.com/watch?v=-FmVCDx_kFw.
20. Ania M. Jastreboff et al., "Tirzepatide Once Weekly for the Treatment of Obesity," *New England Journal of Medicine* 387, no. 3 (2022): 205–16, https://doi.org/10.1056/NEJMoa2206038.
21. Rodriguez et al., "Discontinuation and Reinitiation of Dual-Labeled GLP-1 Receptor Agonists Among U.S. Adults With Overweight or Obesity."
22. Prime Therapeutics, "Prime Continues to Lead Industry on GLP-1 Research."
23. Blue Health Intelligence, *Real-World Trends in GLP-1 Treatment Persistence and Prescribing for Weight Management.*
24. Rodriguez et al., "Discontinuation and Reinitiation of Dual-Labeled GLP-1 Receptor Agonists Among U.S. Adults With Overweight or Obesity."
25. Jason Cohen, "Max MRR: Your Growth Ceiling," A Smart Bear, July 27, 2025, https://longform.asmartbear.com/max-mrr/.
26. App Economy Insights, "Hims & Hers: Surging Telehealth," Substack, How They Make Money, September 24, 2024, https://www.appeconomyinsights.com/p/hims-and-hers-surging-telehealth.

27. HIMS & HERS HEALTH, INC., *Form 10-K For the Fiscal Year Ended December 31, 2024*, Form 10-K (U.S. Securities and Exchange Commission, 2024), https://www.sec.gov/Archives/edgar/data/1773751/000177375125000062/hims-20241231.htm.
28. Author's synthesis based on Mohit Sodhi et al., "Risk of Gastrointestinal Adverse Events Associated With Glucagon-Like Peptide-1 Receptor Agonists for Weight Loss," *JAMA* 330, no. 18 (2023): 1795–97, https://doi.org/10.1001/jama.2023.19574; Rodriguez et al., "Discontinuation and Reinitiation of Dual-Labeled GLP-1 Receptor Agonists Among U.S. Adults With Overweight or Obesity."

Part II

Keeping Your Customers: Lessons from the Outside

CHAPTER 4

THE APPLE PRICING LESSON

In June 2007, Steve Jobs stood on a stage in San Francisco. He held up a phone and said that it was five years ahead of anything else on the market. He priced it at $599.[1] At that price, the iPhone was a luxury toy. It was for tech fans and early adopters who would pay extra to be first. The plan made sense if you thought you were selling a piece of hardware.

In the beginning, sales were decent. Then they stalled. Sixty-eight days after launch, Apple cut the price by $200.[2] Jobs put out a public apology. He told early buyers that "the technology road is bumpy" and offered them a $100 store credit. "We want to do the right thing for our valued iPhone customers," he wrote. "We apologize for disappointing some of you."[3] Those words pointed to the next twenty years of Apple's growth.

Apple had figured out something simple. Each customer was worth more than one sale. The 2.08 billion iPhones now in active use are doorways to a long relationship.[4] By 2022, the App Store had handled $1.1 trillion in customer spending.[5] Every iPhone sold feeds a high-margin services business that now drives most of Apple's profit.

WHERE APPLE ACTUALLY MAKES MONEY

By 2017, Apple's real genius was wallet share. Wallet share is a simple idea: how much money one customer spends with you over time. Apple's services arm pulled in about $30 billion in 2017 at 55% gross margins. That was 13% of the company's total revenue.[6] By 2025, services revenue had grown to $109 billion at 75% gross margins. Services were now 26% of total revenue but produced about half of Apple's gross profit.[7] Hardware margins held flat at 37%.[8]

The 2007 price cut was Apple admitting that the iPhone was a platform, not a luxury toy. Platforms die without volume. Jobs put it plainly: "It benefits both Apple and every iPhone user to get as many new customers as possible in the iPhone *tent*."[9]

But the price cut alone did not make Apple a three-trillion-dollar company; what Apple built *after* the cut did—first market share, then wallet share. Apple launched the App Store in 2008 and later added iCloud, Apple Music, and Apple Pay. Together, those services now generate $109 billion a year at 75% margins.[10]

The hardware opened the door. The services kept people inside. Only after that retention engine was running could Apple charge premium prices for hardware again, because the services revenue justified it. Customers stayed not because they were trapped, but because each new piece of the system delivered ongoing value. Switching costs time, learning, and convenience, not just money.

The pharmaceutical industry is now living through its own version of Apple's first 68 days. GLP-1 medications launched at $1,000 to $1,350 a month.[11] Demand surged. Affordability held it back. By 2025, fewer than 4% of eligible patients were on treatment. The price cut is now underway. Government negotiations, direct-to-consumer channels, and generic pressure are all pushing prices down. Average treatment cost is set to fall by more than half in 2026.[12] The question facing this industry is the same one Apple faced in 2007: What do you build after the price cut so volume becomes retention?

THE ACTUAL COST OF MAKING THESE MEDICATIONS

The gap between the cost of making these drugs and what patients pay creates the opening this chapter examines. Making injectable semaglutide involves the active drug, the inactive ingredients that hold it together, the fill-and-finish work, the packaging, and the injector pen itself. That combination forms the manufacturing cost. A normal generic market would add a fair profit on top of that. That total is the cost-based price. Then there is the market price, what manufacturers actually charge, and the gap between the two is dramatic.

A 2024 study in the Journal of the American Medical Association (JAMA) estimated the cost-based price for injectable semaglutide at $0.89 to $4.73 a month at the standard diabetic dose. Across 12 countries, the actual market price for the same drug ranged from $38 to $354 a month.[13] In the United States, list prices were over $1,300 a month before the recent price cuts. Even at today's lower cash prices, that is a 25- to 100-fold markup over what it costs to make the drug.

The JAMA authors define a fair cost-based price as one that "would be expected in competitive markets that afford manufacturers sustainable returns, while avoiding excessive profit margins."[14] That definition builds in a 10% to 50% profit margin, plus tax and operating expenses. Even on those generous terms, injectable semaglutide could be sold profitably for less than $100 per month.

In Chapter 2, I showed that revenue from injectable semaglutide and tirzepatide may flatten in 2026 as prices fall. But losing revenue is not the same as losing money. Manufacturers and health-system middlemen chose extraction pricing in the U.S. and global markets. There is plenty of margin still inside the system. That margin could fund infrastructure and expand access. The manufacturing economics of GLP-1 medications remain very profitable.

THE AVAILABILITY OF MEDICATIONS IN ORAL FORM

Oral semaglutide and orforglipron medications are now available in the United States. The FDA approved oral semaglutide in late December 2025.[15] Starting doses cost $149 per month, and maintenance doses, during which patients spend most of their treatment time, cost $299 per month.[16] Orforglipron is priced similarly.[17] Both are selling well in their early months on the market. Will daily oral medication options be better for retention than injections for weight loss? We will learn as we go in 2026.

The cost-based price of oral semaglutide is higher than that of the injectable. The estimate is $39 to $72 per month. The pill needs a lot more active drug, because the stomach breaks most of it down before it can be absorbed. The obesity dose is two to three times the diabetic dose; therefore, the obesity pill could have a cost-based price of $75 to $125 a month. At a maintenance market price of $299, the oral protocol squeezes margins compared to the injectables. Manufacturers will still make substantial profits, with gross margins being somewhere between 42% and 70% at obesity doses. But the cushion is smaller. As manufacturers figure out how to improve the medication's absorption, margins will improve again.

GLOBAL PRICING ON THE HORIZON

A second shift in pricing is also underway around the world. American patients have been paying for global drug development for years. In 2024, Wegovy cost $7,400 to $8,400 a year in the United States. The same drug costs about $2,230 in Denmark, $1,680 in Germany, and $1,100 in the United Kingdom.[18] Wealthy European countries pay roughly 15% to 30% of the U.S. net price.

Eli Lilly's CEO, Dave Ricks, has proposed what he calls *one fair price*. Under his plan, developed countries would pay prices set by their wealth relative to the United States.[19] If Germany earns 75% of what the U.S. earns per person, Germans should pay 75% of the U.S. price, not 20%. Applied to today's numbers, that would mean German prices rising by 350%.

In late 2025, Eli Lilly raised the United Kingdom list price of Mounjaro by 170%, from £122 to £330 a month for the highest dose.[20] The reasoning was strategic. U.S. rules, such as the Most-Favored-Nation Order, try to tie American prices to the lowest international prices. If international prices stay low while U.S. prices fall, the company loses margin across the board. Raising international prices defends the reference price.

The cost and coverage picture in this chapter will look different in the UK, Germany, and Canada by 2027. International patients who can afford treatment today may be affected as manufacturers protect their U.S. margins.

THE BEST BUY ALTERNATIVE

Apple's success is rooted in its deep vertical integration, or ownership of as many nodes of the supply chain as possible. They make their own hardware and control their operating system. They built the App Store and earn from everything it sells. Every layer belongs to Apple, so every dollar of services revenue flows back to Apple. But what if you do not own the whole supply chain?

Best Buy built a billion-dollar services business on hardware it did not make. In October 2002, Best Buy bought a small Minneapolis computer repair company called Geek Squad for about $3 million. Robert Stephens had founded Geek Squad in 1994 with $200 and a bicycle. He sent technicians in white shirts and black clip-on ties to fix computers in customers' homes. What Best Buy bought did not bring in much revenue. It was a blueprint for building high-margin services on top of products made by someone else.

Best Buy does not make televisions. Samsung, LG, and Sony do. Best Buy does not make laptops. Apple, HP, and Dell do. Best Buy resells commodity hardware, where margins are compressed by Amazon's price-matching software. Geek Squad gave Best Buy something Amazon could not ship in a box.

The math of commodity retail is unforgiving. Best Buy's overall operating margin has run in the low single digits for most of the last decade, typically 3% to 5%.[21] When Hubert Joly took over as CEO in 2012, services were only about 5% of domestic revenue, yet Joly built his turnaround around them, committing Best Buy to becoming "the preferred authority and destination for technology products, services, and solutions."[22] He treated store labor and Geek Squad as the competitive moat rather than the cost to cut.

In September 2017, Best Buy launched Total Tech Support, a $199 annual subscription giving members unlimited Geek Squad help on any device, no matter where it was bought.[23] By January 2023, the renamed Totaltech program had grown to 5.8 million members, generating roughly $1.2 billion in annual recurring revenue.[24] Best Buy then restructured the offering into three tiers in mid-2023, with the top tier, My Best Buy Total, priced at $179.99 annually.[25] By the end of 2025, Best Buy's blended gross profit rate rose from 22.1% to 22.6%, an improvement the company attributed explicitly to "improved financial performance from services and membership offerings."[26]

Best Buy survived Amazon by adding a service layer that no online competitor could replicate. Amazon can ship a television. Best Buy can mount it on the wall, connect it to the sound system, and answer the call when something stops working on a Sunday night. The service layer turns a single transaction into a relationship.

THE CUSTOMER ACQUISITION COST CRISIS

For digital health companies, the smaller margin forces a tighter business model. Hims & Hers saw its customer acquisition cost (CAC) rise as high as $929 in 2024. CAC is the amount a company spends on marketing to acquire one new customer. That is a 71% jump from $544 in 2021.[27] A $929 CAC made sense when the product was a high-margin injectable at $600 or more a month. At those prices, you earn back the cost of acquisition in a few months.

The oral era stretches this model but does not break it. Patients start at $149 per month for four weeks, then move up to $299 per month in maintenance. At a $929 CAC and a roughly 50% product margin, a company earns about $75 in gross profit per starting-dose month and about $150 per month at maintenance. A patient who stays for 12 months delivers about $1,650 in gross profit. That earns the acquisition cost back with room to spare.

The problem is that patients are not staying on treatment. Every patient acquired at today's CAC who stops before month 12 is a loss. Each extra percentage point of churn deepens the loss. Every dollar spent on acquisition that does not turn into retention is a waste. The only path forward is to lower acquisition costs and grow market share more cheaply, by pushing harder on retention and on wallet share. Apple solved the same problem by turning users into their own marketing channel: word-of-mouth, beautiful design, lock-in across devices, and the social proof of two billion phones. Best Buy solved it by building service relationships that brought customers back.

WAYNE'S CALCULATION

Wayne is caught in two gaps at once. The first is the Cost-and-Coverage gap. He has no insurance. Even if he did, it would not cover GLP-1s for obesity. He is making a monthly choice about whether the medication is worth the money.

The second gap is harder to see. Wayne was paying full price to suffer through side effects no one had prepared him for. His clinic devised an on-and-off dosing pattern for him. No one explained why that pattern made him feel worse. Tirzepatide might have suited him better. Some patients who cannot tolerate semaglutide do well on the dual agonist. But Tirzepatide costs more, and his family doctor did not have the training to troubleshoot with Wayne.

Three months after stopping, his A1c has crept up from 6.2 to 6.3. He has gained back most of the weight he lost. The post-meal fog is worse. He fights to stay awake during afternoon client meetings. He thinks about restarting. The specialty clinic is 40 minutes away, open only during business hours, and has a three-month wait for new patients. He runs the math: close his shop for half a day, reschedule two clients, ask his dispatcher to cover, drive 80 minutes round trip, sit in a waiting room, spend 15 minutes with a doctor who will probably restart the same medication that made him miserable. The math does not work for him.

Digital health companies stepped into this gap with a clear pitch: "We treat obesity. Click here." No three-month wait. No closing the shop. No driving. A text-based intake, sometimes a quick video call, and medication shipped to your door in a day or two. The promise was access itself.

But the gap goes deeper than access. Wayne still does not understand what happened to him. He lost 15 pounds on semaglutide and does not know how. In his mind, the drug was a tool that helped him eat less. So now, off the drug, he should be able to do the same thing through willpower. Cut the carbs. Smaller portions. He still thinks of obesity as a behavior problem that needs a behavior solution.

Wayne can know his health is getting worse and still not restart. He has filed the medication under *a diet aid that did not work for me*, not under *treatment for a chronic disease*. His biology does not care how he files it. Obesity is a problem of how the body controls hunger and energy. GLP-1 medications repair that signaling. When the medication is stopped, the biological pull to regain the weight comes back. The same Wayne who would never stop his blood thinner has stopped his obesity medication, because obesity does not feel to him like that kind of disease.

There is a name for what is happening in his brain. Behavioral economists call it *temporal discounting*: the human tendency to weigh today's costs more heavily than tomorrow's, even when tomorrow's cost is much bigger. The framework comes from the work that earned Daniel Kahneman the Nobel Prize.[28] Wayne's brain compares the cost of $350 this month with the cost of a heart attack in 12 years and decides to skip the medication. The nausea last week is vivid in his memory. The plaque building in his arteries is invisible. Each month's choice to stop feels reasonable on its own. The damage adds up anyway.

TWO TYPES OF GAPS

The Cost-and-Coverage Gap

Recall that the GLP-1 retention problem has two parts. This is the first gap, and the most visible one—the $1,350 monthly price tag, the insurance denials, and the prior authorization paperwork. This is the budget hit that pushed North Carolina's State Health Plan to drop coverage after spending $100 million in a single year.[29] About half of patients stop treatment in real-world settings because of cost and coverage barriers.[30] This barrier is real, and market forces are now closing it. TrumpRx negotiations, Medicare pricing pressure, generic competition, and direct-to-consumer channels are all pushing prices down. The pills at $149 to $299 a month are in a different price category than the $1,350 injectables. Manufacturers, payers, and policymakers are working to close this gap.

The Retention System Gap

This is the second gap. It is where the other half of the people who stop treatment live.[31] We know what *good* looks like because specialty obesity programs have shown it. At Vanderbilt's academic weight loss center, patients get a full team:[32]

- Doctors trained in obesity medicine
- Dietitians
- Mental health counselors
- Exercise physiologists
- Integrated pharmacy systems with refill reminders
- Direct messaging to providers

The program also takes cost out of the equation. Patients pay nothing for medications, visits, or services.[33]

Even there, half of the patients had stopped treatment by 12 months. The median stay was 10.7 months.[34] Compare that to the 64.8% who stop in the general insurance population.[35] The specialty model improves retention by about 15 percentage points. It also proves that even with optimal support and zero cost, half of the patients leave within a year.

The model cannot scale. Vanderbilt enrolled 2,306 patients over about three years. They did this at a single academic medical center with shared electronic records, a built-in pharmacy, patient portals, and easy referral pathways.[36] Serving 126 million eligible Americans at that rate would take more than 50,000 equivalent programs. The infrastructure for that exists at only a handful of places. Wayne could not make this kind of program work for his life, even if it were free, because no one's time is free.

In 2005, A. G. Lafley, then the CEO of Procter & Gamble, gave us a useful framework for what was happening.[37] He called it the *moments of truth*. The first moment of truth is when a shopper picks one product over another on the store shelf. The second moment of truth is what happens when they use it at home. If the product fails at the second moment, no amount of advertising or shelf placement at the first moment will save the business. The shopper will not buy it again.

The second moment of truth is the retention system gap. Clinical trials showed patients losing 15% to 20% of their body weight on these medications. That created huge demand. That was a powerful first moment of truth for GLP-1s. The second moment of truth has been a letdown. Two-thirds of patients in the real world stop within a year. They get the medication without the trial infrastructure that made the trials work. The gap between what the drug can do and what it actually does in their lives often decides whether they stay. Optimizing prescription volume optimizes for the first moment. The retention gap is a second moment problem. As Lafley understood, you cannot fix a second moment failure by working harder on the first.

WHAT ABOUT THE APP STORE AND GEEK SQUAD?

The GLP-1 market needs its own version of the App Store and Geek Squad to address why patients actually quit:

- The side effects no one prepared them for
- The food confusion when their tastes change overnight
- The absence of coaching when things get hard
- The loneliness of figuring it out alone

The retention layer should do what good clinicians have always done: turn a prescription into an ongoing relationship.

The drug companies cannot solo-build the App Store and Geek Squad, but they have the strongest incentive of all to figure out how to keep patients from abandoning their hardware. A drug company cannot prescribe its own medication without a few arms-length layers. A company that profits from a prescription cannot also be the one making prescribing decisions, not without crossing basic medical ethics and most likely federal anti-kickback rules.

When Eli Lilly and Pfizer launched their direct-to-consumer platforms, Senators Dick Durbin, Bernie Sanders, Elizabeth Warren, and Peter Welch sent letters asking whether the setups were "intended to steer patients toward particular medications" and created "the potential for inappropriate prescribing."[38] Regulators are watching.

LillyDirect and similar programs, therefore, function as pricing and distribution programs rather than integrated clinical platforms. Eli Lilly can set the price at $349 per month. They can partner with Walmart for pharmacy pickup and Amazon for home delivery, but the clinical assessment, the prescribing decision, and the ongoing care must come from independent providers. For prescribing, LillyDirect partners with Form Health, knownwell, 9amHealth, and Ro. These are telehealth companies that make their own clinical calls, are not paid to prescribe Eli Lilly's medications, and do not pay Eli Lilly for referrals.

This is the opposite of Apple's model. Apple built a platform that kept customers as Apple customers, no matter which app they used. The Best Buy model is the relevant parallel for anyone who wants to build retention infrastructure in GLP-1 care. Best Buy built a service business on products made by other companies. Digital health companies do not synthesize semaglutide or tirzepatide. But they can build a service business on top of medications made by Novo Nordisk and Eli Lilly.

Some of the most successful apps in the App Store are not made by Apple. Spotify, for example, outperforms Apple Music.[39] The platforms that win in obesity care will build what manufacturers, traditional clinics, and the current crop of digital platforms cannot or will not. The most obvious candidate is a clinically sound, commercially viable retention system that helps patients succeed.

ENDNOTES

1. James Mitchell, *The Apple iPhone*, Teaching case no. UV1228 (Darden Business Publishing, University of Virginia, 2010).
2. Mitchell, *The Apple iPhone.*
3. Ibid.
4. Robert A. Lee, "Apple Statistics 2025: Revenue, Devices & Services," *SQ Magazine*, May 22, 2025, https://sqmagazine.co.uk/apple-statistics/.
5. Juliette Caminade and Jonathan Borck, *The Continued Growth and Resilience of Apple's App Store Ecosystem* (2023), https://www.apple.com/newsroom/pdfs/the-continued-growth-and-resilience-of-apples-app-store-ecosystem.pdf.
6. Apple Inc., *Form 10-K for the Fiscal Year Ended September 30, 2017* (U.S. Securities and Exchange Commission, 2017), https://www.sec.gov/Archives/edgar/data/320193/000032019317000070/a10-k20179302017.htm.
7. "The $4 Trillion Fortress: A Deep-Dive Analysis of Apple Inc. (AAPL) in 2025," PredictStreet, December 23, 2025, https://markets.financialcontent.com/wral/article/predictstreet-2025-12-23-the-4-trillion-fortress-a-deep-dive-analysis-of-apple-inc-aapl-in-2025.
8. Apple Inc, *Form 10-K for the Fiscal Year Ended September 27, 2025* (U.S. Securities and Exchange Commission, n.d.), accessed December 29, 2025, https://www.sec.gov/Archives/edgar/data/320193/000032019325000079/aapl-20250927.htm.
9. Mitchell, *The Apple iPhone.*
10. PredictStreet, "The $4 Trillion Fortress: A Deep-Dive Analysis of Apple Inc. (AAPL) in 2025."
11. Steven D. Pearson et al., "Affordable Access to GLP-1 Obesity Medications: Strategies to Guide Market Action and Policy Solutions in the U.S.," *Journal of Comparative Effectiveness Research* 14, no. 9 (2025): e250083, https://doi.org/10.57264/cer-2025-0083.
12. Author's calculation based on TrumpRx negotiated prices and Medicare projections; see The White House, "Fact Sheet: President Donald J. Trump Announces Major Developments in Bringing Most-Favored-Nation Pricing to American Patients," The White House, November 6, 2025, https://www.whitehouse.gov/fact-sheets/2025/11/fact-sheet-president-donald-j-trump-announces-major-developments-in-bringing-most-favored-nation-pricing-to-american-patients/.
13. Melissa J. Barber et al., "Estimated Sustainable Cost-Based Prices for Diabetes Medicines," *JAMA Network Open* 7, no. 3 (2024): e243474, https://doi.org/10.1001/jamanetworkopen.2024.3474.
14. Barber et al., "Estimated Sustainable Cost-Based Prices for Diabetes Medicines."
15. Tom Murphy et al., "Trump Unveils Deal to Expand Coverage and Lower Costs on Obesity Drugs," *Magnolia Tribune*, November 6, 2025, https://magnoliatribune.com/2025/11/06/trump-unveils-deal-to-expand-coverage-and-lower-costs-on-obesity-drugs/.

16. "GLP-1 Pill Information," Wegovy® (Novo Nordisk), accessed December 29, 2025, https://www.wegovy.com/about-wegovy/the-wegovy-pill.html.
17. The White House, "Fact Sheet."
18. Pearson et al., "Affordable Access to GLP-1 Obesity Medications."
19. *Dave Ricks, CEO of Eli Lilly, on GLP-1s and the Business of Pharma*, directed by Stripe, 2025, https://www.youtube.com/watch?v=-FmVCDx_kFw.
20. Lauren Almeida, "Eli Lilly Ramps up UK Price of Weight Loss Jab Mounjaro after Trump Demands," Business, *The Guardian*, August 14, 2025, https://www.theguardian.com/business/2025/aug/14/eli-lilly-uk-price-weight-loss-jab-mounjaro-trump.
21. John R. Wells and Gabriel Ellsworth, "Reinventing Best Buy," HBS No. 716–455 (Boston: Harvard Business School Publishing, rev. May 4, 2018), Exhibit 2.
22. Hubert Joly, remarks at Best Buy analyst and investor day, New York, November 13, 2012; cited in Wells and Ellsworth, "Reinventing Best Buy," p. 4.
23. Wells and Ellsworth, "Reinventing Best Buy," p. 14 (citing Best Buy investor day, September 19, 2017).
24. Melissa Repko, "Best Buy doubles down on membership program as sales cool," CNBC, May 11, 2023, citing Best Buy CEO Corie Barry on Q1 FY24 earnings call.
25. Best Buy, "Best Buy unveils My Best Buy Memberships™," press release, May 11, 2023.
26. Best Buy Co., Inc., Form 10-K for fiscal year ended February 1, 2025 (filed March 2025), Management's Discussion and Analysis section.
27. DrugPatentWatch, "The Rise of Telehealth Companies Like Ro and Hims & Hers: How Direct-to-Consumer Telehealth Redefined the Pharmaceutical Value Chain," DrugPatentWatch, October 5, 2025, https://www.drugpatentwatch.com/blog/novel-pharmaceutical-strategies-and-business-models-the-rise-of-telehealth-companies-like-ro-and-hims-hers/.
28. George Loewenstein and Drazen Prelec, "Anomalies in Intertemporal Choice: Evidence and an Interpretation*," *The Quarterly Journal of Economics* 107, no. 2 (1992): 573–97, https://doi.org/10.2307/2118482.
29. Alan Goforth, "North Carolina Ends Coverage of New Weight Loss Drugs for 750,000 State Employees," *BenefitsPRO*, May 17, 2024.
30. Patricia J. Rodriguez et al., "Discontinuation and Reinitiation of Dual-Labeled GLP-1 Receptor Agonists Among U.S. Adults With Overweight or Obesity," *JAMA Network Open* 8, no. 1 (2025): e2457349, https://doi.org/10.1001/jamanetworkopen.2024.57349.
31. Hamlet Gasoyan et al., "Reasons for Discontinuation of Obesity Pharmacotherapy With Semaglutide or Tirzepatide in Clinical Practice," *Obesity* 33, no. 12 (2025): 2296–303, https://doi.org/10.1002/oby.70058.
32. Jason M. Samuels et al., "Real-World Titration, Persistence & Weight Loss of Semaglutide and Tirzepatide in an Academic Obesity Clinic," *Diabetes, Obesity and Metabolism* 27, no. 11 (2025): 6200–209, https://doi.org/10.1111/dom.70004.

33. Samuels et al., "Real-World Titration, Persistence & Weight Loss of Semaglutide and Tirzepatide in an Academic Obesity Clinic."
34. Ibid.
35. Rodriguez et al., "Discontinuation and Reinitiation of Dual-Labeled GLP-1 Receptor Agonists Among U.S. Adults With Overweight or Obesity."
36. Samuels et al., "Real-World Titration, Persistence & Weight Loss of Semaglutide and Tirzepatide in an Academic Obesity Clinic."
37. Shep Hyken, "The New Moment of Truth in Business," Forbes, accessed May 8, 2026, https://www.forbes.com/sites/shephyken/2016/04/09/new-moment-of-truth-in-business/.
38. "Durbin Leads Senators in Demanding Answers from Pfizer, Eli Lilly on New Telehealth Platforms Amid Concerns of Inappropriate Prescribing | U.S. Senator Dick Durbin of Illinois," accessed May 8, 2026, https://www.durbin.senate.gov/newsroom/press-releases/durbin-leads-senators-in-demanding-answers-from-pfizer-eli-lilly-on-new-telehealth-platforms-amid-concerns-of-inappropriate-prescribing.
39. Zhixuan Huang, "A Comparative Analysis of Spotify and Apple Music: Revenue Structures, Profit Models, and Strategic Positioning," *Advances in Economics, Management and Political Sciences* 223 (October 2025): 156–65, https://doi.org/10.54254/2754-1169/2025.GL27752.

CHAPTER 5

THE TICKETMASTER TRAP

By the middle of 2022, pharmacies could not keep Ozempic in stock.[1] The molecule, semaglutide, was approved for type 2 diabetes, but physicians across the country were prescribing it off-label for weight loss. Prescription volumes overwhelmed Novo Nordisk's manufacturing capacity. Between 2019 and 2024, GLP-1 prescriptions spiked 587%.[2] Ozempic became the top-selling drug by revenue in Canada, generating billions in annual pharmacy sales despite constrained access.[3]

GLP-1s were social-media-fueled cultural phenomena, and every major news outlet was running weekly coverage of *the skinny shot*. The FDA declared a semaglutide shortage in March 2022, followed by a tirzepatide shortage in December 2022.[4] Patients with diabetes and those seeking weight loss could not access their treatments the usual way.

Manufacturing capacity for the GLP-1 market was built for the diabetes-only era. When the obesity-driven demand surged, the major bottleneck was in making the auto-injector pens, each of which held a month or more of medication. Peptide synthesis was scalable, but pen assembly was not. Pen assembly lines take years to build, and manufacturers did not build enough of them.[5]

Enter compounding pharmacies. In Chapter 2, we learned that compounding pharmacies are allowed to make *essentially copies* of FDA-approved drugs if those drugs appear on the official shortage list.[6] This rule was intended as a safety valve during emergencies. It is a good way to keep patients in treatment when primary supply chains fail. In the GLP-1 supply crisis, Sections 503A and 503B were the narrow channels that widened into an ocean-sized parallel market.

Patients flocked to lower-cost treatments from suppliers they learned about on Facebook groups. Chief among them was a new crop of digital health platforms, led by Hims & Hers, which irreversibly disrupted the market for weight-loss medications. Simultaneously, a more mature gray market was telling us exactly how this would go.

In November 2022, 14 million Taylor Swift fans logged into Ticketmaster at the same time. They were hoping to grab seats for the Eras Tour. Most watched progress bars crawl for hours. Many were kicked out of the queue. Those who made it through found that tickets listed at $49 had vanished. They were replaced by *platinum* seats priced at $449 or more.[7]

Two years later, Oasis fans in the UK lived through the same story. Tickets advertised at £148 surged to £350 through *dynamic pricing* while fans waited in digital queues. The outrage was immediate because Ticketmaster controlled an estimated 70% of the ticketing and live events market. Ticketmaster's 2024 revenues reached $23.2 billion. The company could weather the backlash and didn't change course.[8]

Ticketmaster creates scarcity by locking up venues through exclusive contracts. Then it demands high prices from the most willing-to-pay buyers. Fans cannot go elsewhere because of this near monopoly on venues, so they try to scalp tickets online. But the company also profits from the resale market because it owns the resale platforms. Scarcity is the business model. And it works for them because Ticketmaster has monopolistic power and owns the entire value chain from primary sale through resale.

GLP-1 manufacturers tried to leverage the same scarcity dynamic as Ticketmaster. They set prices high and did not rush to cover supply shocks. They created the conditions for a legal secondary market. But unlike Ticketmaster, pharmaceutical companies do not own the secondary market because they do not control compounding pharmacies. Patients seeking obesity treatment in 2022, finding never-ending backorders, also turned to the secondary market. Many of these patients did not perceive or care about the difference between compounded semaglutide and Wegovy, especially when their neighborhood pharmacy's shelves were empty, but the compounded version could be delivered to their doorstep tomorrow.

Ticketmaster's scarcity model traps and exploits value. Pharmaceutical companies tried the same, but it did not work. Patients learned to shop based on price. They lost confidence in brand names and stopped treating FDA clearance as something worth paying for. By the time supply normalized, the perception of branded weight loss medications was undermined by a legitimate, booming secondary market that, as far as patients could tell, did the same thing for a fraction of the cost. This is the *Ticketmaster trap*.

THE REGULATORY SQUEEZE

Once a drug is removed from the shortage list, it is considered *commercially available*. The legal exception allowing compounders to make *essentially copies* is revoked. The telehealth platforms that built their business models on compounded GLP-1s are grappling with an existential choice: transition to branded products, find alternative formulations that qualify as *significantly different* under Section 503A, or exit the market. Figure 5.1 depicts the timing of the three U.S. government actions in eight months that closed the legal window for compounded GLP-1s in the U.S., but enforcement has been slow to materialize.

Many compounders tried to bypass the ban by adding ingredients such as Vitamin B12 or changing delivery forms. The FDA explicitly warned that compounders cannot rely on "mere pretextual differences" to evade federal law. Adding B12 alone does not automatically make a drug *not a copy*. The prescriber must specifically explain why the addition produces a significant difference for that specific patient.[9]

On February 21, 2025, when the FDA announced the end of the semaglutide shortage, Hims & Hers stock dropped 25% in a single trading day.[10] The company had built significant value, with $589.1 million in quarterly revenue and 50.1% year-over-year growth.[11] But the market instantly repriced them. Access arbitrage closed. They were not valued as a durable care platform. They were valued as a temporary access play.

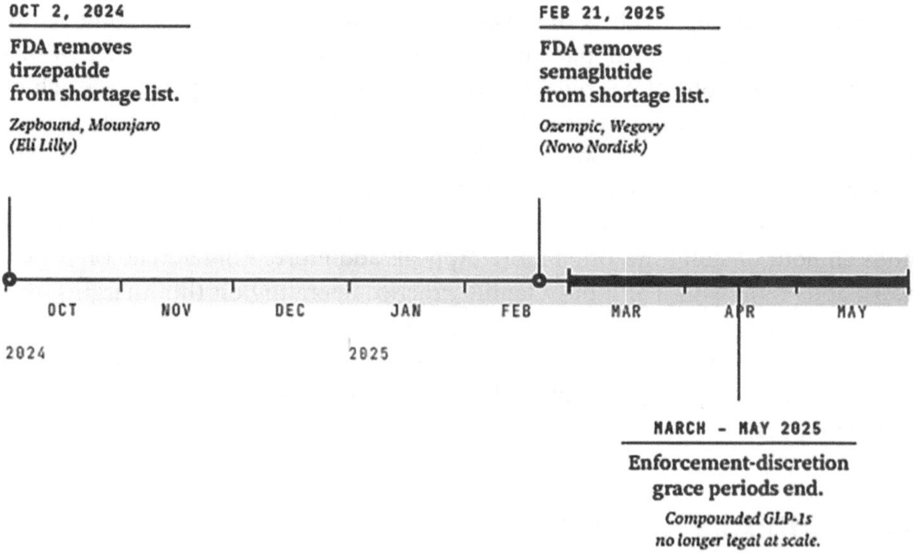

Figure 5.1 The GLP-1 regulatory squeeze.

Sources: Nathan A. Beaver and David L. Rosen, "GLP-1 Drugs: FDA Removes Lilly's Zepbound® and Mounjaro® (Tirzepatide Injection) from Its Drug Shortage List," Foley & Lardner LLP, October 7, 2024, foley.com/insights/publications/2024/10/glp-1-drugs-fda-removes-lillys-zepbound-and-mounjaro-tirzepatide-injection-from-its-drug-shortage-list/; Nathan A. Beaver and David L. Rosen, "GLP-1 Drugs: FDA Removes Semaglutide from the Drug Shortage List," Foley & Lardner LLP, February 25, 2025, foley.com/insights/publications/2025/02/glp-1-drugs-fda-removes-semaglutide-from-drug-shortage-list/; FDA, "FDA Clarifies Policies for Compounders as National GLP-1 Supply Begins to Stabilize."

Yet despite the legal closure, enforcement has been very slow to materialize. At the very end of 2025, the FDA was finally warning compounders to stop selling compounded semaglutide and tirzepatide.[12] At the same time, and perhaps not coincidentally, both Novo Nordisk and Eli Lilly started slowly lowering their prices for uninsured patients in the U.S.

THE PRESCRIPTION ECONOMICS PROBLEM

The compounding market did not vanish when supply normalized. The economics of obesity prescribing in primary care makes the gray market structurally appealing, even now. When a family physician sees a patient for obesity, the assessment is the product. In the United States, a primary care visit generates revenue between \$23 and \$221, depending on complexity and payer.[13] That is fifteen minutes—questions, history, exam, decision, notes—that is the billable event.

But the work does not stop there. GLP-1 prescriptions almost always trigger prior authorization, which is the insurance company requiring the clinic to fill out paperwork before it will pay for the drug. My office handles every step of that paperwork, and none of it is billable. We document failed alternatives, record biometrics, cite clinical evidence, and fill out a 17-field form. We wait on hold to confirm receipt. We follow up two weeks later when the request sits unreviewed. We field pharmacy calls about dosing. Each task is unpaid.

The assessment fee was supposed to cover fifteen minutes. Prior authorization adds an hour of staff time, often more. Appeals add more. Annual renewal paperwork adds more still. For a busy family practice operating on thin margins, this administrative tail makes GLP-1 prescriptions economically punishing to write. My colleagues in primary care have not stopped caring about their patients with obesity. They have stopped being able to afford treating them inside their traditional practices.

THE PRIMARY CARE MYTH

Sarah had been on Wegovy for six weeks and lost five pounds. It was covered by her insurance with a \$50 copay. Then her employer emailed to say they were dropping coverage for obesity medications due to budget constraints. Sarah either had to figure out how to pay \$1,329 a month (the price in 2024) out of pocket or else stop taking the medication.

My appointment with Sarah ran ten minutes long because we needed 20 minutes to prepare an appeal strategy. We didn't get to talk about her palate changes or her energy levels. A family doctor quickly learns which conditions grind the gears of their practice and which ones do not. GLP-1 prescriptions fall squarely into the first category.

Market projections assume this will solve itself. TD Securities projects global GLP-1 sales reaching $139 billion by 2030, but that forecast depends on "meaningful uptake of weight loss drugs in the primary care setting."[14] ICER (Institute for Clinical and Economic Review) makes the same assumption. It argues that *open prescribing* by primary care is the only strategy that *maximizes access* given the specialist shortage.[15] ICER is an independent U.S. nonprofit that evaluates cost-effectiveness and shapes how payers think about coverage decisions. When ICER says primary care must lead, payers listen.

The problem is that primary care cannot lead. The channel is already overwhelmed. Primary care physicians make up 31% of the physician workforce but absorb 46% of all medical visits.[16] They handle 500 to 577 million visits every year. The average panel size is more than 2,000 patients per physician.[17] Every extra minute spent on prior authorization for Sarah is a minute not available for another patient's chest pain, depression screening, or diabetes follow-up.

The workforce is also getting smaller. Nearly half of primary care physicians are 55 years of age or older.[18] Fewer nurse practitioners and physician associates are choosing to enter the specialty. Projections suggest a shortage of 20,000 to 40,000 primary care physicians by 2036.[19] The channel that market analysts assume will absorb the obesity epidemic is shrinking and aging out of the workforce at the same time.

The $139 billion projection depends on a delivery system that is already at capacity, economically punished for writing these prescriptions, and getting smaller every year. This is the gap between market forecasts and clinical reality. Analysts model demand, but they forget to model who is supposed to meet it.

THE CASH-PAY BYPASS

Most commercially insured patients could not get coverage for obesity medications anyway, even if their prior authorization process was perfect. They were pushed to the cash-paying market, where they perceive more options and more help. Ro, Hims & Hers, and similar companies built their GLP-1 businesses around direct-to-consumer, cash-pay models. No prior authorization forms. No appeals. No middlemen. The patient pays and then receives the medication, usually at their door. The entire administrative apparatus that makes prescribing obesity medication miserable for primary care physicians did not exist for this crop of digital health platforms. Ro has since introduced insurance navigation tools to help patients access coverage,[20] an evolution I return to in Chapter 11.

For patients who cannot get primary care appointments or who are underinsured, a direct cash-pay model removes real barriers. But it requires a margin to fund. A digital health company that spends $929 to acquire a patient who pays only $100 for a consultation loses money on day one.[21] The only way to make the unit economics work is to capture revenue beyond the visit. That is why these companies built pharmacies and took control of dispensing. Margins on compounded obesity medications could be so high because the list prices of branded medications were, by comparison, out of reach. Compounded semaglutide for $299 only seemed like a great deal because Wegovy was charging an absurd $1329.

After the shortage was resolved, and now during the era of price compression, compounding platforms have to navigate a much tighter regulatory squeeze while trying to maintain the low-friction cash-pay model that appeals to patients. These companies will still exist in the post-compounding world because prior authorization is fraught, and primary care doctors aren't realizing the upside of obesity treatment in their practices. The structural incentives that made compounding initially appealing remain largely intact.

SARAH'S BRAND-TRUST PROBLEM

Sarah is a fact finder. She read about compounding pharmacies, understood the rules, and recognized the risks. She felt that staying on treatment mattered more than staying on a specific brand. She found a telehealth platform advertising compounded semaglutide for $299 per month and made the switch.

With it, Sarah's relationship with the Wegovy brand broke. She realized she had been paying for a brand premium that did not seem worth it to her. The compounded version kept her losing weight, it cost a fraction of the price, and it was actually available when Wegovy was not. When the shortage was eventually resolved, I offered Sarah the chance to return to the branded medication while staying under my care. But she still had no coverage, and she declined. She chose to continue with compounded semaglutide.

When patients discovered they could get compounded semaglutide for a quarter of the list price, they felt exploited by manufacturers who used scarcity pricing during an epidemic, and by insurance companies that arbitrarily distinguished between diabetes and obesity. By mid-2024, the compounding market was serving an estimated one to two million patients and generating $3 to $4 billion in annual revenue. A KFF (Kaiser Family Foundation) Health News headline captured the scale: "Why Millions Are Trying FDA-Authorized Alternatives to Big Pharma's Weight Loss Drugs."[22]

Sarah photographed a vial of her compounded semaglutide and texted it to a friend who was considering treatment. "Same thing, a quarter of the price, and you can actually get it." Her friend signed up the next week. The supply failure did not just create a temporary access problem; it permanently altered how patients perceive the relationship between brand, molecule, and value. Trust, once broken, is very difficult to rebuild.

THE CANADIAN CRYSTAL BALL

The U.S. market stays protected by patents until at least December 2031. But, in 2019, Novo Nordisk missed a routine maintenance fee of about $450 in Canadian dollars (CAD) on the core compound patent for semaglutide in Canada.[23] On January 4, 2026, Novo Nordisk's regulatory data exclusivity on semaglutide ended. This is a protection layer that blocks generic makers from relying on the brand's clinical trial data. Multiple generic manufacturers filed applications for their own semaglutide with Health Canada as early as 2024. By January 2026, nine submissions from at least five companies were under review.[24] Then Novo Nordisk did something unexpected.

On December 22, 2025, two weeks before data exclusivity expired, Health Canada approved two new drug names for semaglutide: Plosbrio and Poviztra.[25] If they come to market, they will be made by Novo Nordisk using the same manufacturing lines as their higher-priced brand sisters. The only differences are the name and packaging. Health Canada confirmed explicitly that these are not generic products and have no connection to the generic review process.[26]

Kate Hanna, a spokesperson for Novo Nordisk Canada, confirmed that the company is considering competing in the generic market with these products.[27] The strategy would let Novo Nordisk keep Ozempic and Wegovy at premium pricing while setting Plosbrio and Poviztra close to whatever the generics eventually charge. Two brands at two price points, serving the entire market. This is the Ticketmaster lesson, fully learned: *If you cannot prevent the secondary market, own it yourself.*

The Authorized Generic Playbook

The pharmaceutical industry has a name for this strategy: the *authorized generic.* An authorized generic is the exact same drug as the brand, made on the brand's production line, but packaged with a generic label. Because it is sold under the original new drug application rather than a separate generic application, the brand company can launch it without waiting for regulatory approval of a generic competitor.[28]

Pfizer wrote the playbook for this in 2011, when Lipitor, then the best-selling drug in the world, lost patent protection. Rather than watch generic competitors capture the entire market, Pfizer partnered with Watson Pharmaceuticals to launch an authorized generic of atorvastatin on the exact same day the first independent generic hit the market.[29] The result: Pfizer captured about 70% of generic revenue during the first 180 days and retained 30% of the U.S. market share even after multiple competitors entered.[30] The U.S. Federal Trade Commission has since quantified the damage to independent generics. When an authorized generic competes during the first-filing generic's 180-day exclusivity period, the first-filer's revenue runs 40% to 52% below what it would be without that competition, and stays 53% to 62% below over the following 30 months.[31]

When patients switch from brand to generic, their prescriptions are filled with whatever sits on the pharmacy shelf. If the brand company's authorized generic is sitting next to the independent generic, both at similar prices, the brand company captures half the volume that would otherwise go to competitors. The per-unit margin is lower, but their total revenue is higher.

Novo Nordisk is applying the same logic preemptively. Instead of waiting for generics to erode their market and then responding, they have positioned Plosbrio and Poviztra to be on pharmacy shelves before any independent generic can.

The Regulatory Delay Advantage

I have been preparing clinically for the practice-changing effects of more affordable semaglutide for over a year. Patients ask all the time about when their monthly medication expenses might drop. I do not know exactly when the first generic semaglutide will be given to one of my patients. One of them will let me know when they go to pick up their medication and find themselves a few hundred dollars better off than expected.

Semaglutide sits between two kinds of medicine. Small-molecule drugs like aspirin are built in a lab through chemical reactions. Biologics are complex proteins made by living cells, the same way insulin is brewed inside genetically engineered yeast. Novo Nordisk produces Ozempic and Wegovy using the biologic method. Yeast cells, modified to act as tiny factories, secrete the semaglutide peptide, which the company then purifies for clinical use.[32] The generic companies are proposing a different route entirely. They want to build the same 31-amino-acid peptide through chemistry alone, stitching it together one amino acid at a time. The molecule that comes out is supposed to be identical to the original. The manufacturing path that produces it is fundamentally different, which is why Health Canada cannot apply its usual generic approval framework to these applications.

Health Canada requires proof that these manufacturing differences do not affect clinical performance, a more demanding standard than typical generic approvals.[33] The Canadian Generic Pharmaceutical Association has noted that without published guidance on what these applications should include, each manufacturer submits, receives requests for clarification, and resubmits in a prolonged back-and-forth.[34]

The gap between generic filing and approval gives Novo Nordisk time to establish pharmacy relationships, build supply chain presence, and become the default substitution option before any independent generic reaches the shelf. First-mover advantage in generic markets is substantial. Research on the Lipitor transition showed that early entrants captured market share that persisted for years after competitors entered the market.[35]

Canadian pricing regulations allow generic medications to be priced at 35% of the brand reference price.[36] For semaglutide, that means roughly $80 to $110 CAD per month instead of $300 or more. At these prices, more patients will enter the market. There will be downward price pressure on compounders, which are rare in Canada to begin with, and insurers will reconsider coverage for weight-loss medications at these prices.

The cross-border pressure from U.S. patients will be immediate. Florida has received federal approval for a Section 804 importation program, a legal pathway for American patients to access Canadian medications.[37] American patients will see Canadian neighbors accessing the same treatment for a fraction of the price. Faced with the compounding market and coming generic competition, manufacturers have deployed two distinct strategies: (1) direct-to-consumer pricing and (2) gray-market retatrutide.

In Brand Defense

Eli Lilly has filed lawsuits against multiple telehealth and digital health companies offering compounded tirzepatide.[38] Novo Nordisk has filed at least 21 lawsuits against companies that produce and sell purported copies of semaglutide.[39] Both companies have petitioned the FDA to restrict compounding on the argument that the drugs present *demonstrable difficulties* that make them unsuitable for the process.

This is like Ticketmaster suing scalpers instead of fixing the ticketing system. It is legally defensible and strategically necessary to protect intellectual property (IP). But lawsuits do not recapture the millions of patients who have already learned to access treatment outside the brand ecosystem.

BRIDGE BEHAVIOR: DIRECT-TO-CONSUMER PRICING

LillyDirect and Novo Nordisk's NovoCare Pharmacy, which began offering Wegovy at $499 per month in March 2025, work with partners to deliver lower-cost medications to self-paying patients.[40] These are bridge behavior programs—the manufacturers' response to the unexpected price-elasticity of their generational molecules. Eli Lilly explicitly refuses to partner with any company that compounds GLP-1 medications through LillyDirect, a policy that excludes Hims & Hers from the partnership entirely, despite their massive presence in telehealth obesity treatment.

The anti-compounding stance serves multiple purposes. It protects Eli Lilly's IP, maintains quality control over the medications patients receive, and creates a bright line separating LillyDirect from the regulatory gray zone where compounders operate. When the FDA's February 2025 declaration ended the semaglutide shortage and triggered deadlines for compounders to cease production, the companies aligned with LillyDirect were insulated from the disruption.

The policy also means Eli Lilly does not work with some of the largest patient acquisition engines in the market. The clinical partners Eli Lilly selected for LillyDirect (discussed in Chapter 4) are more clinically specialized and less aggressive in customer acquisition. The conflict-of-interest constraint and the anti-compounding policy together tell us that Eli Lilly and Novo Nordisk are playing the long game. They care about the reputation of their medications and how they are delivered. If only their initial pricing decisions better reflected this.

In April 2026, Medicare announced a pilot program covering Zepbound and Wegovy for obesity at a standardized monthly price of $245.[41] This represented a 75% to 80% reduction from market prices. It was recognition that the prior pricing model could not scale to support a public health intervention for a disease this consequential.

The drug manufacturers accepted price compression in the U.S. cash-paying market because the alternative was losing the entire segment to compounding. But accepting lower margins domestically created a different problem. How do you maintain global revenue growth when your largest market is compressing?

Their response was to raise prices everywhere else. That strategy recreates in international markets the exact problem they are trying to escape in the United States. UK patients paying £330 per month will do the same math Sarah did. German patients facing 350% increases will seek the same workarounds. The volume capture problem does not disappear; it just moves abroad. Manufacturers are closing the cost gap in the United States while widening it internationally at the same time, and patients in global markets will respond exactly the way American patients did, by finding another way in.

The Ubiquity of Gray-Market Retatrutide

The breach in brand trust created by extractive pricing and supply shortages did not just drive patients to compounded versions of approved medications. It opened the door for highly valuable pipeline medications to be accessed illegally before they received FDA approval for human use.[42]

Retatrutide is Eli Lilly's *triple-agonist* targeting GLP-1, GIP, and glucagon receptors. In Phase 2 trials that tested whether a drug would work in a small group of patients, retatrutide demonstrated up to 24.2% weight loss over 48 weeks, outperforming every currently approved option.[43] The drug is still in Phase 3 trials, the larger and longer studies that are the final step before FDA approval.[44] At this time, it has no FDA approval and has not been authorized for human use outside of controlled clinical studies. And yet, what online suppliers are calling *retatrutide* is readily available for purchase on social media for $100 to $200 per month.[45]

The progression was very fast. Once the market became comfortable with compounded semaglutide, accepting that the gray-market version was *similar enough* to the FDA-approved version, the transition to retatrutide required no additional mental leap. Biohackers and optimization-focused consumers began calling it *GLP-3*, the next-generation upgrade.[46] Rather than wait for FDA approval (expected around 2026 or 2027), they went straight to a supply chain operating entirely outside regulatory oversight. Manufacturers located mostly in China produce freeze-dried peptide powders labeled *for research use only* or *not for human consumption*. These substances are shipped directly to U.S. consumers or through middlemen, bypassing every safety and sterility standard the FDA exists to enforce.[47] A *BMJ* investigation documented sellers on TikTok and Facebook marketing counterfeit retatrutide. One patient was offered a box of generic retatrutide by a personal trainer who claimed it came from a "Swiss lab."[48]

Safety data for authentic retatrutide exists only within controlled trials.[49] Quality assurance for products purchased through unregulated channels is absent. Counterfeits may contain no active ingredient, and they may contain contaminants that pose immediate harm. Consumers have no way to tell the difference.

The FDA has explicitly warned that retatrutide cannot legally be used in compounding because it is not a component of any FDA-approved drug.[50] Eli Lilly has stated that anyone selling retatrutide is breaking the law and has taken legal action against online sellers.[51]

None of this has meaningfully slowed the market. I have had patients ask me about peptides they found on Instagram. The conversation is always the same. They show me a screenshot. I ask what they know about where it was made. They do not know. I ask what they know about who is prescribing it. They do not know. I explain what *for research use only* means on a label: no one in the supply chain has a legal or professional obligation to the person injecting it. Some patients hear me, and some do not. I have no way to compete with an Instagram advertisement offering *GLP-3* for $150 a month, because I am not selling a product. I am selling an inconvenient truth: the FDA-approved options cost more and carry actual prescriber accountability. The gray market has trained patients to associate that accountability with friction rather than with safety and value.

Manufacturers set prices that patients perceived as exploitative and allowed supply shortages to persist for nearly two years despite having the capacity to resolve them. Then, when they demonstrated through their actions that patient access was subordinate to margin protection, they created the conditions for this market to emerge. Patients who had been priced out, denied coverage, or left waiting through shortages learned that the system was not designed to serve them. And once that pathway was normalized, it did not stop at FDA-approved molecules; it extended to any intervention that promised better outcomes, regardless of legal status or safety profile.

THE ESCAPE ROUTE

Retention is earned, not demanded. Scarcity pricing works when the seller owns the entire value chain, but fails catastrophically when the seller does not. Pharmaceutical manufacturers assumed their patent exclusivity was equivalent to Ticketmaster's venue contracts. It was not. A venue contract is enforced by the physical reality that a concert happens in one place at one time. A drug patent is enforced by laws with loopholes for emergency shortages, by foreign jurisdictions with different patent regimes, and by a regulatory regime that lets underground peptide manufacturers ship freeze-dried powder directly to consumers. The exclusivity was always more fragile than the pricing strategy assumed.

ENDNOTES

1. American Society of Health-System Pharmacists, "Drug Shortage Detail: Semaglutide Injection," ASHP Drug Shortages Resource Center, March 5, 2025, https://www.ashp.org/Drug-Shortages/Current-Shortages/Drug-Shortage-Detail.aspx?id=813.
2. *Obesity and GLP-1 Drugs: A Claims-Based Analysis*, White Paper (FAIR Health, Inc., 2025), https://s3.amazonaws.com/media2.fairhealth.org/whitepaper/asset/Obesity%20and%20GLP-1%20Drugs%20-%20A%20FAIR%20Health%20White%20Paper.pdf.
3. Chris Hannay, "Canada Will Be a Launching Pad in the Global Race for Generic Ozempic," *The Globe and Mail*, January 30, 2026.
4. Velimir Altabas et al., "Addressing the Shortage of GLP-1 RA and Dual GIP/GLP-1 RA-Based Therapies—A Systematic Review," *Diabetology* 6, no. 6 (2025): 52, https://doi.org/10.3390/diabetology6060052.
5. American Society of Health-System Pharmacists, "Drug Shortage Detail."
6. "FDA Clarifies Policies for Compounders as National GLP-1 Supply Begins to Stabilize," U.S. Food and Drug Administration (FDA), FDA, April 28, 2025, https://www.fda.gov/drugs/drug-safety-and-availability/fda-clarifies-policies-compounders-national-glp-1-supply-begins-stabilize.
7. Normand Turgeon and Yany Grégoire, "The Modern Ticketing Industry: Ticketmaster's Past, Present, and Beyond," *International Journal of Case Studies in Management* 22, no. 5 (2024).
8. Turgeon and Grégoire, "The Modern Ticketing Industry: Ticketmaster's Past, Present, and Beyond."
9. FDA, "FDA Clarifies Policies for Compounders as National GLP-1 Supply Begins to Stabilize."
10. Heather Landi, "FDA Declares Semaglutide Shortage over, Spelling End to Compounded GLP-1 Market, for Now," February 21, 2025, https://www.fiercehealthcare.com/health-tech/fda-declares-semaglutide-shortage-over-spelling-end-compounded-glp-1-market.
11. "Hims & Hers Health, Inc. (HIMS): Business Model Canvas," DCF Modeling, December 2025, https://dcfmodeling.com/products/hims-business-model-canvas.
12. Brian J. Malkin and Elizabeth A. Siemer, "FDA and Novo Nordisk Warned of GLP-1 Telehealth Compounding Takedown. What's Next?," Pharmacy Times, March 26, 2026, https://www.pharmacytimes.com/view/fda-and-novo-nordisk-warned-of-glp-1-telehealth-compounding-take-down-what-s-next-.
13. "Search the Physician Fee Schedule," CMS.Gov, accessed December 30, 2025, https://www.cms.gov/medicare/physician-fee-schedule/search.
14. Michael Nedelcovych et al., "GLP-1 Market: The Pipeline Expands—AHEAD OF THE CURVE®," TD Securities, March 10, 2025, https://www.tdsecurities.com/ca/en/glp1-market-the-pipeline-expands.

15. Steven D. Pearson et al., "Affordable Access to GLP-1 Obesity Medications: Strategies to Guide Market Action and Policy Solutions in the U.S.," *Journal of Comparative Effectiveness Research* 14, no. 9 (2025): e250083, https://doi.org/10.57264/cer-2025-0083.
16. Brian Antono et al., *Primary Care in the U.S.: A Chartbook of Facts and Statistics* (Robert Graham Centre, 2021), https://www.graham-center.org/content/dam/rgc/documents/publications-reports/reports/PrimaryCareChartbook2021.pdf.
17. American Medical Association, *Future of Health Case Study: Omada Health* (American Medical Association, n.d.).
18. "U.S. Physician Workforce Data Dashboard," AAMC, accessed May 8, 2026, https://www.aamc.org/data-reports/report/us-physician-workforce-data-dashboard.
19. *The Complexities of Physician Supply and Demand: Projections from 2021 to 2036* (Association of American Medical Colleges, 2024), https://www.aamc.org/media/75231/download.
20. "Ro Launches the GLP-1 Insurance Coverage Checker," Ro, August 13, 2024, https://ro.co/press/glp1-insurance-coverage-checker/.
21. "The Unbundling of the Apothecary: How Vertically Integrated Telehealth Is Dismantling the Pharmaceutical Value Chain," DrugPatentWatch, May 5, 2025, https://www.drugpatentwatch.com/blog/novel-pharmaceutical-strategies-and-business-models-the-rise-of-telehealth-companies-like-ro-and-hims-hers/.
22. Arthur Allen Zenda Oona, "Why Millions Are Trying FDA-Authorized Alternatives to Big Pharma's Weight Loss Drugs," *KFF Health News*, July 23, 2024, https://kffhealthnews.org/health-industry/glp1-compounding-pharmacies-wegovy-zepbound-copycat-drugs-shortages/.
23. "The Semaglutide Story: Highlighting the Need to Maintain Patent Protection in Canada," Brunet & Co, July 1, 2025, https://www.brunetco.com/the-semaglutide-story-highlighting-the-need-to-maintain-patent-protection-in-canada/.
24. "Apotex Wins Tentative FDA Approval for Generic Ozempic, Drug Makers Await Health Canada Decisions," *The Globe and Mail*, April 12, 2026, https://www.theglobeandmail.com/business/economy/article-apotex-fda-approval-generic-ozempic-drug-health-canada-decisions/.
25. "Novo Nordisk Prepares New Cheaper Version of Ozempic as Generics Face Delays," *The Globe and Mail*, January 5, 2026, https://www.theglobeandmail.com/canada/article-ozempic-cheaper-version-novo-nordisk-health-canada-generics/.
26. *The Globe and Mail*, "Novo Nordisk Prepares New Cheaper Version of Ozempic as Generics Face Delays."
27. Ibid.
28. Definitions, 21 CFR § 314.3 Code of Federal Regulations (2026).
29. Pfizer, *Form 10-K for the Fiscal Year Ended December 31, 2011*, Form 10-K (Washington, DC, 2011), https://www.sec.gov/Archives/edgar/data/78003/000119312512085703/d278590d10k.htm.
30. Duff Wilson, "Facing Generic Lipitor Rivals, Pfizer Battles to Protect Its Cash Cow," CNBC, November 30, 2011, https://www.cnbc.com/2011/11/30/facing-generic-lipitor-rivals-pfizer-battles-to-protect-its-cash-cow.html.

31. Federal Trade Commission, "Authorized Generic Drugs: Short-Term Effects and Long-Term Impact: A Report of the Federal Trade Commission" (Washington, DC: Federal Trade Commission, August 2011), https://www.ftc.gov/sites/default/files/documents/reports/authorized-generic-drugs-short-term-effects-and-long-term-impact-report-federal-trade-commission/authorized-generic-drugs-short-term-effects-and-long-term-impact-report-federal-trade-commission.pdf.
32. Jesper Lau, Paw Bloch, Lauge Schäffer, Ingrid Pettersson, Jane Spetzler, Jacob Kofoed, Kjeld Madsen, Lotte Bjerre Knudsen, James McGuire, Dorte Bjerre Steensgaard, Hanne Müller Strauss, Dorte X. Gram, Sven Munk Knudsen, Flemming Seier Nielsen, Patrick Thygesen, Steffen Reedtz-Runge, and Thomas Kruse. "Discovery of the Once-Weekly Glucagon-Like Peptide-1 (GLP-1) Analogue Semaglutide." *Journal of Medicinal Chemistry* 58, no. 18 (2015): 7370–380. https://doi.org/10.1021/acs.jmedchem.5b00726.
33. Health Canada, "Canada Becomes the First G7 Country to Approve a Generic Version of Semaglutide," news releases, April 28, 2026, https://www.canada.ca/en/health-canada/news/2026/04/canada-becomes-the-first-g7-country-to-approve-a-generic-version-of-semaglutide.html.
34. *The Globe and Mail*, "Novo Nordisk Prepares New Cheaper Version of Ozempic as Generics Face Delays."
35. J. Daniel McGeeney et al., "Measuring the First Mover Advantage in U.S. Biosimilar Markets," *Value in Health* 28, no. 12 (2025): 1814–25, https://doi.org/10.1016/j.jval.2025.07.011.
36. "Generic Drugs," Pan-Canadian Pharmaceutical Alliance, accessed May 8, 2026, https://www.pcpacanada.ca/generic-drug-framework.
37. Brunet & Co., "The Semaglutide Story: Highlighting the Need to Maintain Patent Protection in Canada."
38. Dae Lee and Lucas Morgan, "GLP-1 Litigation Escalates: What Pharmacies and Telemedicine Providers Need to Know," Buchanan Ingersoll & Rooney PC, April 25, 2025, https://www.bipc.com/glp-1-litigation-escalates-what-pharmacies-and-telemedicine-providers-need-to-know.
39. Arthur Allen, "Why Millions Are Trying FDA-Authorized Alternatives to Big Pharma's Weight Loss Drugs," *KFF Health News*, July 23, 2024, https://kffhealthnews.org/news/article/glp1-compounding-pharmacies-wegovy-zepbound-copycat-drugs-shortages/.
40. "LillyDirect and Walmart Pharmacy Launch First Retail Pick-up Option with Direct-to-Consumer Pricing for Zepbound | Eli Lilly and Company," Lilly, October 29, 2025, https://investor.lilly.com/news-releases/news-release-details/lillydirect-and-walmart-pharmacy-launch-first-retail-pick-option; "Novo Nordisk Introduces NovoCare® Pharmacy, Lowering Cost of All Doses of FDA-Approved Wegovy® (Semaglutide) to $499 per Month and Offering Easy Home Delivery for Cash-Paying Patients," PR Newswire, March 5, 2025, https://www.prnewswire.com/news-releases/novo-nordisk-introduces-novocare-pharmacy-lowering-cost-of-all-doses-of-fda-approved-wegovy-semaglutide-to-499-per-month-and-offering-easy-home-delivery-for-cash-paying-patients-302392874.html.

41. "Weight-Loss Drugs Enter a New Phase of 'Price-for-Volume': Consumerization Trends Accelerate, and Lower Prices Will Stimulate Significant Demand Release," December 8, 2025, https://www.moomoo.com/news/post/62586834/weight-loss-drugs-enter-a-new-phase-of-price-for.
42. Bloomberg, host, *The Booming Business of Chinese Peptides*, Odd Lots, December 19, 2025, 48:48, https://www.youtube.com/watch?v=QErGuO-mtfc.
43. Ania M. Jastreboff et al., "Triple–Hormone-Receptor Agonist Retatrutide for Obesity—A Phase 2 Trial," *New England Journal of Medicine* 389, no. 6 (2023): 514–26, https://doi.org/10.1056/NEJMoa2301972.
44. Kate Bowie, "Weight Loss Jabs: Eli Lilly Cracks down on Fake Drugs Being Sold on TikTok and Facebook," *BMJ* 391 (October 2025): r2202, https://doi.org/10.1136/bmj.r2202.
45. Bloomberg, *The Booming Business of Chinese Peptides.*
46. Ibid.
47. Ibid.
48. Bowie, "Weight Loss Jabs."
49. Ibid.
50. Bloomberg, *The Booming Business of Chinese Peptides.*
51. Bowie, "Weight Loss Jabs."

CHAPTER 6

PELOTON WAS NOT SELLING BIKES

In September 2020, Peloton posted its first-ever quarterly profit.[1] By January 2021, the company had built a market capitalization approaching $50 billion on the back of $2,000 exercise bikes during the pandemic. Demand outstripped supply, and customers were waiting months for delivery. Executives responded by committing $420 million to acquire commercial fitness equipment maker Precor, and another $400 million to build a U.S. factory in Ohio.[2] They were betting on at-home fitness as the permanent default.

Sixteen months later, Peloton halted all bike production. They canceled the contract to build the Ohio factory, and thousands of jobs were eliminated.[3] The stock, which peaked at $167.42 in January 2021, collapsed to under $10 by mid-2022. This was a $47 billion collapse in shareholder value.[4] Throughout all of it, Peloton's subscription retention rate held above 92%.[5]

Peloton almost failed because it believed it sold spin bikes. The company's very name was a clue about what customers actually wanted. A *peloton* is a tight-knit group of cyclists riding and racing together in a pack. Peloton was in the business of shared, competitive fitness experiences that customers could access without leaving their living rooms. It was never just about the bike.

Many digital health companies in the weight loss space are making the same mistake. They believe they just sell medication. Patients are not there only for semaglutide or tirzepatide. They are there for what becomes possible with sustainable weight loss: eating well without mental distress, moving more easily, managing weight-related disease, better sleep, improved fertility, and more. The medications enable transformation, but they don't define it.

In Peloton terms, the medication is the bike. What the patient gets after the medication arrives at their door is the subscription. The subscription business saved Peloton while hardware nearly tanked it. The real-world retention statistics in obesity medication treatment are so dismal because the industry expected it could install the bike in every home (i.e., sell the medication to willing patients) and let the magic unfold. It turns out patients have to actually *ride* the bike, so to speak. And, as with Peloton, they need more than a monthly delivery to make that happen.

HIGH RETENTION, WRONG METRIC

Before its initial public offering in 2019, Peloton reported a 12-month retention rate of 95%.[6] This was remarkable in the fitness industry, where gym memberships typically see annual churn rates (the percentage of customers who cancel) of 27% to 29%. A survey by William Blair found that 96% of Peloton owners would recommend the product to a friend.[7] At the peak of the pandemic, the average subscriber did 26 workouts a month. Users engaged with the platform nearly every day.[8]

These are among the highest engagement and retention metrics in consumer technology. Peloton created a product that improved people's fitness habits and built deep loyalty. In 2020, Peloton generated $1.8 billion in revenue. Subscription gross margins, the profit percentage left after subtracting production costs, reached 56.8%. Hardware gross margins were 45.3%.[9] But the company's strategy, its capital allocation, and its supply chain investments were all oriented around hardware production and delivery. When pandemic demand spiked, Peloton did not invest in subscriber success infrastructure. It invested in making more bikes, faster.

By mid-2021, quarterly hardware sales had dropped over 50% from their peak. Hardware gross margins fell from above 30% to 12%. The company was sitting on $1.5 billion in unsold inventory. Bicycles and treadmills sat on cargo ships and in warehouses, the result of a misread demand.[10]

Meanwhile, subscription revenue kept growing. Subscription gross profit overtook hardware gross profit for the first time by June 2021.[11] The recurring revenue stream, built on ongoing customer success, remained healthy even as the hardware business cratered.

THE $50 BILLION MANUFACTURING BET

Novo Nordisk acquired Catalent for $16.5 billion to bring fill-finish production in-house. Fill-finish is the process of putting drugs into their final vials and injection pens.[12] Eli Lilly has committed over $50 billion to manufacturing infrastructure, including a $5.3 billion facility in Indiana.[13] The bet is that lower prices will unlock enormous pent-up demand, and that capacity will be the rate-limiter for capturing it.

The bet is correct as far as it goes. There is pent-up demand, and price compression will reveal it. Chapter 2 showed the $84 billion gap between actual and potential revenue at a 15% share benchmark, and Chapter 5 showed how the shortage-era supply constraints sent millions of patients to compounders, who then did not return. Building capacity is necessary.

It is also not sufficient, and the Peloton story tells us why. Peloton built more bikes and ended up with $1.5 billion in unsold inventory because it misread what customers were really buying. Pharma is now building more factories to serve a retention system that cannot retain its existing patients. Expanding capacity without solving this problem is the Peloton mistake. The wallet-share problem from Chapter 3 does not go away because the factory got bigger. Long-term value in chronic disease comes from patients staying well, which means staying on treatment; therefore, the infrastructure around the prescription has to work. But how do we get patients back on the bike?

HOW PELOTON SAVED ITSELF

Peloton survived its near-death experience through a complete change of direction. By late 2025, subscription revenue represented roughly 70% of total revenue, up from approximately 20% before the pandemic.[14]

The shift required rethinking customer acquisition entirely. Customer acquisition cost dropped from roughly $500 per subscriber to approximately $130. The drop was achieved mostly through business-to-business partnerships that created what the company calls *sampling surfaces*, places where potential customers could try the product before buying.[15] Rather than spending marketing dollars to convince consumers to buy expensive hardware from afar, Peloton placed the hardware where people would naturally encounter it. They literally put their buyers on the bike.

In October 2022, Peloton installed bikes in nearly all 5,400 Hilton-branded hotels across the United States.[16] Business travelers experience the product during their stay. A portion of them end up purchasing bikes for their homes or subscribing to the app without Peloton spending traditional acquisition dollars. The hotel bikes function as mini trial periods and reveal the potential for transformation.

Peloton hired Peter Stern as CEO in January 2025 to run what it now understands itself to be: a subscription company. Stern cofounded Apple Fitness+ and spent 25 years building subscription businesses at Time Warner Cable, Ford, and Apple.[17] Even the secondary market reinforces this strategic shift. Used Pelotons flood resale sites. Bikes that used to retail for $2,000 now sell for $400 to $600 online. Rather than fighting this loss of new-bike sales, Peloton embraced it. Someone who buys a used bike from a neighbor still pays $44 monthly for content access.

The company no longer cares who owns the hardware. It cares who subscribes to the service, and it optimizes for engagement metrics that predict long-term retention: workout frequency, class completion rates, and community participation.

WHAT MADE THE PELOTON SUBSCRIPTION STICK

Peloton built specific mechanisms that turned exercise from an obligation into a daily ritual experienced in community. The instructors functioned as minor celebrities rather than fitness coaches. They shared personal struggles, posted frequently on social media, and cultivated followings that often exceeded those of Peloton's own brand channels. Users described their relationship with instructors as feeling like a *second family* or *friends*. These were one-sided bonds where the rider felt like they knew the instructor, even though the instructor did not know them. These para-social relationships make canceling the subscription feel like abandoning a true friend.[18]

The platform engineered an atmosphere of *belonging* through community architecture. Tags like #PelotonMoms, #BlackLivesMatter, and #PelotonTeachers allowed users to self-organize into micro-communities. Digital high-fives provided real-time validation. Instructors gave shout-outs for milestones. The Century Ride, a customer's 100th class, came with badges and recognition that made exercise into a ritual.[19] The software created the social dynamics of an in-person class without requiring anyone to leave their living room.

Content production matched streaming service quality. State-of-the-art studios in New York and London produced visually engaging, music-driven classes that felt like TV shows rather than workout videos. There were classes with live DJs and genre-specific rides. By 2020, noncycling workouts accounted for 36% of all fitness sessions.[20] The subscription delivered value whether you owned the bike or not.

The platform turned progress into a game you did not want to quit. Real-time leaderboards let competitive riders race strangers. Auto-follow tracked performance over time, building streaks that felt costly to break. Detailed metrics fed the drive to track your own numbers. Riders knew their average output, their personal records, their improvement curves. Some maintained subscriptions just to preserve their progress history.[21]

The subscription-first strategy broke the link between subscription value and owning the bike. A $12.99 per month digital-only tier made Peloton competitive with Netflix. Customers could access the same celebrity instructors and high-quality content with or without equipment. Apps for Apple Watch, Fire TV, and other platforms followed and made the subscription work wherever customers were.[22]

WEIGHTWATCHERS WAS WATCHING

In 2023, WeightWatchers watched its subscriber base collapse from 5 million in 2020 to 3.5 million in 2022. They saw the GLP-1 wave approaching and made what looked like the right move.[23]

CEO Sima Sistani said, "Most U.S. doctors aren't trained in obesity medication, and there's not a clear, safe, trusted way for people to understand whether they should be on these medications. WeightWatchers can be that source."[24] The company had 60 years of behavioral support infrastructure. GLP-1 medications require behavioral support to work long term. The combination seemed obvious.

In March 2023, WeightWatchers acquired Sequence, a telehealth company specializing in chronic weight management, for $132 million.[25] By December, they launched WeightWatchers Clinic, a subscription offering GLP-1 access combined with coaching for $83 per month.[26] The strategy mirrored what Peloton eventually learned. The hardware, or in this case the prescription, is the entry point. The ongoing relationship is the business.

By mid-2024, WeightWatchers Clinic had 81,000 subscribers against a target of 140,000 to 160,000. Total company revenue declined 10.9% quarter over quarter. The stock fell 89.5% for the calendar year.[27] Oprah Winfrey left the board.[28]

What went wrong was that WeightWatchers correctly diagnosed the problem but built the wrong infrastructure for it. They had the heritage. They had brand recognition. They acquired telehealth capability. But they underestimated the distance between diet-based weight loss and chronic disease treatment.

WeightWatchers' existing infrastructure was designed for people trying to eat less. Their entire system of points, weigh-ins, and accountability groups assumed the problem could be boiled down to overconsumption. The solution, in their model, was restriction. Patients on GLP-1 medications often face the opposite challenge. Treatment suppresses appetite so effectively that many struggle to eat *enough*. Foods they have loved for decades become unappealing. They need to learn how to fuel their bodies when hunger signals are dampened and unreliable. WeightWatchers had no content for this. Their coaches were not trained for it. Their app was not built around it. The Sequence acquisition gave WeightWatchers the capability to prescribe. It did not give them the ability to help patients actually succeed on these medications.

The company also lacked the clinical infrastructure to catch problems early, and this is the gap the medicine punishes hardest. When a patient hits severe nausea at a dose increase, someone needs to intervene within days, not weeks. WeightWatchers' model was not designed for the dose-adjustment timeline of injectable medications, where a bad week at the wrong dose can permanently sour a patient on treatment.

The acquisition itself created friction. Employees felt the company was "minimizing the importance of behavioral support" and going in the opposite direction.[29] The internal culture clash between Sequence's clinical telehealth model and WeightWatchers' community-based behavioral model never resolved into a coherent patient experience.

Peloton had bikes and eventually realized they needed to build subscription infrastructure around them. WeightWatchers had subscription infrastructure but discovered that GLP-1 support requires fundamentally different content, touchpoints, and clinical expertise. The behavioral support infrastructure that patients on obesity medications need must be built intentionally, from first principles. It has to be designed around the specific clinical reality of what these medications do to appetite, food preferences, and the daily experience of eating.

WHAT DRIVES DISCONTINUATION?

The first six months are where treatment lives or dies. In my practice, this is the stretch I pay the most attention to, and the research confirms what I see in the exam room. Side effects drive 21% of discontinuation in the first three months, compared with only 8.7% of later discontinuations.[30] The dropout curve is steepest at the beginning, when side effects are most intense, and the benefits have not yet materialized.

Gastrointestinal side effects (nausea, vomiting, diarrhea, and constipation) vary in timing, severity, and duration between patients. Some experience mild nausea for a few days after each dose increase. Others face weeks of severe symptoms. The same dose that one patient tolerates may easily leave another unable to eat. This variability demands individualized response, not standardized protocols.

Side effects by themselves are not the reason patients quit. Patients with moderate or severe gastrointestinal side effects are only 19% more likely to discontinue, and most of these side effects respond well to simple interventions.[31] The problem is that those side effects have to come to the attention of a clinician, or a system that can act on them within days.

What patients too often get is a system that operates reactively. They start medication. They experience side effects. Then they wait weeks for their next appointment. If they mention the problems, adjustments might happen. If they do not mention them, it is usually because they assume this is normal, or do not want to seem difficult, or cannot reach the clinic. Sometimes, they feel they deserve to suffer. What patients need is proactive check-ins, fast dose adjustments, and a clinician or coach who catches trouble before it becomes prolonged silent suffering and dropout.

First impressions do matter. Patients who experience severe gastrointestinal side effects are significantly less likely to ever try medication again once they stop.[32] I have had patients who tried a GLP-1 once, had a miserable two weeks on a dose that was too high, and refused to touch any of these medications even years later. The clinical cost of a poorly managed first month is hard to recover.

Among those who make it past three months, cost is the most common reason for stopping. Side effects still matter at all phases, but cost becomes increasingly important over time. The type of insurance matters enormously. Patients with Medicare or Medicaid were far more likely to cite cost as their reason for stopping, at 61% and 76.5%, respectively, compared with 43% for those with private insurance.[33]

When cost barriers come down, retention improves. The Vanderbilt obesity clinic mentioned in Chapter 4, where patients paid nothing out of pocket, saw only 14% discontinuation at three months compared with rates above 30% in the general population.[34] Cost is not the only thing that the clinic gets right. Clinical flexibility matters too. A separate analysis found that 25% of patients needed to switch medications to stay on treatment at all.[35] Weight loss itself also predicts retention. Analysis of 125,474 patients found that for every 1% reduction in body weight from baseline, there was a 3.3% lower chance of discontinuing the medication.[36]

WHAT *BELONGING* LOOKS LIKE IN PRACTICE

A lot of clinicians can prescribe obesity medications. The factor that determines whether a patient stays on treatment is what happens over the next six months to a year. My patients have to believe me when I tell them it will get better. They have to believe me when I tell them I am helping them stay away from danger, and that I will let them know when some of the discomfort they are experiencing, or the plateau they have hit, is not normal. They trust me to guide them through to an unknown place. I take that trust seriously, and I am front and center for that journey for a lot of people. My experience is that when I show up that way, consistently, the willpower and the loyalty follow.

My patients are extraordinarily loyal. Not because I have created any cult of personality, but because I have shown up for them and cared about their long-term success. They can feel the difference between true concern and a system built to extract a few hundred dollars from them and move on. The consequences for my practice economics are favorable. Acquisition is not something I need to invest in. I invest in relationships, and the referral flywheel does the acquisition for me. Growth is not fast by any measure, but it is durable.

Obesity treatment should feel like showing up for a class you do not want to miss. I believe in milestone celebrations for navigating the first plateau, for retaining muscle mass, and for graciously handling snide comments from colleagues about their changing body. My favorite moments to celebrate with patients are the little ones. Sarah casually mentioned in one of our visits that she was able to cross her legs comfortably for the first time in years. I stopped her. "What does that mean for you?" "It means I can attend a friend's birthday party without stressing about where I am going to sit." It means belonging. It means there is a spot for her in the peloton. I invited her to share her win during our weekly group sessions. The other patients flooded the screen with clapping and heart emojis. They held her accomplishment as sacred. When she needs it, they will remind her that these changes in function matter more than any change in form.

Patients vary considerably in their needs and in what motivates them. Some want data and metrics. Some want encouragement and reassurance. Some want to be left alone until something goes wrong. Peloton lets its users choose. Sustained behavior change requires an infrastructure that makes people want to stay engaged. Doctor's orders are a fiction in chronic disease. Peloton did not succeed by telling people to get on bikes. It succeeded by making the ongoing relationship valuable enough that people showed up even when it was hard, without coercion.

The product is not the prescription. It is the ongoing relationship that makes enduring weight loss possible. Peloton's subscription revenue now represents roughly 70% of total revenue because the company understands this.[37] Pharmaceutical executives who measure success by new prescription volume are celebrating bike sales and ignoring whether anyone is riding.

And the support infrastructure must match the clinical reality. WeightWatchers had decades of behavioral support experience. None of it transferred. Their entire system assumed the problem was overconsumption. GLP-1 patients often face the opposite problem. You cannot graft chronic disease support onto a diet-culture infrastructure. The graft will not take.

If you are building an obesity treatment infrastructure, build it from first principles. Design for the specific clinical reality of these medications, not for a general wellness concept. Build for retention from day one, not as an afterthought once acquisition stalls. Part III will show you how. The companies that do this will own the market, just like Peloton owns experiential at-home fitness.

ENDNOTES

1. Kimberly Chin, "Peloton Posts First-Ever Profit as Pandemic Speeds Sales," Business, *Wall Street Journal*, September 10, 2020, https://www.wsj.com/articles/peloton-posts-first-ever-profit-as-pandemic-speeds-sales-11599776415.
2. Joshua Foster and Ryan Cheng, *Peloton Interactive Inc.: A Push to Keep Users Pedalling*, no. W35254 (Ivey Publishing, Ivey Business School, Western University, 2024).
3. David Wood and Cam Buchan, *Peloton Interactive, Inc.: The Rough Road to Turnaround*, no. W32687 (Ivey Publishing, Ivey Business School, Western University, 2023).
4. Suraj Srinivasan et al., *Peloton Interactive (A)*, nos. 9-323–005 (Harvard Business School, 2025); Frank T. Rothaermel, *Peloton Interactive, Inc.*, MHE-FTR-071 (McGraw Hill Education, 2022); Robert J. Dolan, *Peloton Interactive, Inc. (C): Post the Pandemic Boom*, nos. 9-523–044 (Harvard Business School, 2022).
5. Len Sherman, *How Peloton Built the Foundation for Enduring Success (A)*, no. CU274 (Columbia Business School, 2020).
6. "Peloton's Growth, Decline and Comeback," Growthcurve, September 19, 2025, https://growthcurve.co/pelotons-growth-strategy.
7. E. Scott Mayfield, *Valuing Peloton*, nos. 9-220–060 (Harvard Business School, 2021).
8. Foster and Cheng, *Peloton Interactive Inc.: A Push to Keep Users Pedalling.*
9. Sherman, *How Peloton Built the Foundation for Enduring Success (A).*
10. Dolan, *Peloton Interactive, Inc. (C): Post the Pandemic Boom.*
11. Foster and Cheng, *Peloton Interactive Inc.: A Push to Keep Users Pedalling.*
12. Joseph L. Badaracco et al., "Market Dynamics and Moral Dilemmas: Novo Nordisk's Weight-Loss Drugs," *Harvard Business School Case 324-114*, July 2024.
13. Alex Card, "GLP-1 Drugs Lead Big Pharma into the Direct-to-Consumer Market," Definitive Healthcare, September 6, 2024, https://www.definitivehc.com/blog/glp1-direct-to-customer-investment.
14. Garima Singh, "Case Study: Peloton Faced Slowing Growth—Their Hardware-as-a-Service Model Changed Everything," Circuly, December 12, 2025, https://www.circuly.io/blog/how-peloton-built-a-business-around-hardware-as-a-service; Foster and Cheng, *Peloton Interactive Inc.: A Push to Keep Users Pedalling.*
15. Growth curve, "Peloton's Growth, Decline and Comeback."
16. "Hilton and Peloton Team Up to Enhance the Travel Wellness Experience," Peloton Interactive, Inc., October 3, 2022, https://investor.onepeloton.com/news-releases/news-release-details/hilton-and-peloton-team-enhance-travel-wellness-experience/.
17. "Peloton Appoints Peter Stern as CEO and President," Peloton Interactive, Inc., October 31, 2024, https://investor.onepeloton.com/news-releases/news-release-details/peloton-appoints-peter-stern-ceo-and-president/.
18. Meghan Murray, *Best Self or Best Company? Peloton Searches for a Voice*, no. UV7898 (University of Virginia Darden School Foundation, 2019), https://www.ssrn.com/abstract=3682608.

19. "Peloton's Subscription Playbook Selling More Than Just a Bike," Rajiv Gopinath, May 16, 2025, https://www.rajivgopinath.com/blogs/next-gen-media-and-marketing/the-subscription-economy-and-rentership-culture/the-shift-from-ownership-to-access/pelotons-subscription-playbook-selling-more-than-just-a-bike.
20. Murray, *Best Self or Best Company?*
21. Rajiv Gopinath, "Peloton's Subscription Playbook Selling More Than Just a Bike."
22. "The Peloton Pivot," SBI Growth, January 6, 2025, https://sbigrowth.com/insights/the-peloton-pivot.
23. Ram Subramanian, *WeightWatchers International: The Ozempic Pivot*, no. W43451 (Ivey Publishing, Ivey Business School, Western University, 2025).
24. Nicole Goodkind, "Sima Sistani Says Its Time for WeightWatchers to Embrace Ozempic. Will Its Users Agree?," CNN, November 28, 2023, https://www.cnn.com/2023/11/28/business/sima-sistani-risk-taker.
25. "WeightWatchers to Acquire Sequence, a Digital Health Platform for Clinical Weight Management," Weight Watchers, March 6, 2023, https://corporate.ww.com/news/news-details/2023/WeightWatchers-to-Acquire-Sequence-a-Digital-Health-Platform-for-Clinical-Weight-Management/default.aspx.
26. Nathaniel Meyersohn, "WeightWatchers Launches a New Membership Plan for Ozempic Customers," CNN Business, December 14, 2023, https://www.cnn.com/2023/12/14/business/weightwatchers-ozempic-weight-loss.
27. Subramanian, *WeightWatchers International: The Ozempic Pivot*, 1.
28. Ibid., 5.
29. Ibid., 7.
30. Hamlet Gasoyan et al., "Reasons for Discontinuation of Obesity Pharmacotherapy With Semaglutide or Tirzepatide in Clinical Practice," *Obesity* 33, no. 12 (2025): 2296–303, https://doi.org/10.1002/oby.70058.
31. Patricia J. Rodriguez et al., "Discontinuation and Reinitiation of Dual-Labeled GLP-1 Receptor Agonists Among U.S. Adults With Overweight or Obesity," *JAMA Network Open* 8, no. 1 (2025): e2457349, https://doi.org/10.1001/jamanetworkopen.2024.57349.
32. Rodriguez et al., "Discontinuation and Reinitiation of Dual-Labeled GLP-1 Receptor Agonists Among U.S. Adults With Overweight or Obesity."
33. Gasoyan et al., "Reasons for Discontinuation of Obesity Pharmacotherapy With Semaglutide or Tirzepatide in Clinical Practice."
34. Jason M. Samuels et al., "Real-World Titration, Persistence & Weight Loss of Semaglutide and Tirzepatide in an Academic Obesity Clinic," *Diabetes, Obesity and Metabolism* 27, no. 11 (2025): 6200–209, https://doi.org/10.1111/dom.70004.
35. Gasoyan et al., "Reasons for Discontinuation of Obesity Pharmacotherapy With Semaglutide or Tirzepatide in Clinical Practice."
36. Rodriguez et al., "Discontinuation and Reinitiation of Dual-Labeled GLP-1 Receptor Agonists Among U.S. Adults With Overweight or Obesity."
37. Singh, "Case Study: Peloton Faced Slowing Growth—Their Hardware-as-a-Service Model Changed Everything."

CHAPTER 7

FITBIT: DATA WITHOUT INTERPRETATION

Years ago, Wayne's fitness tracker caught a rapid, irregular heart rate. He asked his doctor about it, and she sent him to the emergency department. The heart tracing at the hospital confirmed a new diagnosis of atrial fibrillation, a condition that increases his risk of stroke and heart failure. The watch provided a signal, and the doctor interpreted its meaning. That was the best-case deployment of a wearable: a single, clear signal, read by someone who could confirm and communicate its meaning. For patients who like their wearables, the data gives them agency that would otherwise show up as anxiety.

Fast-forward to now. Wayne is on a beta blocker and an anticoagulant for his atrial fibrillation. His heart rate still fluctuates because the arrhythmia does that even when treated. He still has the watch. He knows it could show him something. But when the number jumps, he doesn't know whether to be worried, whether to take his pulse, whether to call someone, or whether to just breathe. He doesn't want to overreact by going to the hospital, and his cardiology follow-up is four months out; so, he stops checking. Sometimes in healthcare, to borrow from the late Notorious B.I.G., more data really does create more problems.[1]

DATA WITHOUT A STORY

Early consumer wearables, like the Fitbit wristband, detected data such as heart rate, step count, and sleep score. These measurements have cultural reference points in North America. We have heard of *10,000 steps per day*, just like we have heard of *an apple a day*. In this sense, wearable consumers may feel some comfort with the interpretation of these numbers. Some perceive value in having them available in real time, but for many, the novelty wears off.

GLP-1 medicine pushes us into unfamiliar territory. Patients can feel very full on few calories, so if you ask them if they're fueling well enough, they insist that they are. But if they actually keep a food journal, many are shocked to learn they are eating far fewer calories than is sustainable in the long term. It will contribute to medication drop-off because they begin to feel tired, unwell, and unmotivated. Their hunger signals, previously very powerful, aren't coming across. This requires careful monitoring, especially in the first year of treatment.

Continuous glucose monitors are medical devices approved for use in people with diabetes. I also use them in people without diabetes in my practice, but I don't care just about the average glucose. I care about the volatility of the tracing, the persistence of elevated glucose after meals, how patients respond to certain meal combinations, and whether they experience meaningful patterns that correlate with their appetite, energy, or sleep. I interpret continuous glucose data manually with patients because the automatic reports I get from the monitor companies presume that I am treating diabetes when I am actually trying to prevent the disease by using an entirely different interpretation layer. I also capture body composition data, habit trackers, menstrual calendars, and the typical diagnostics.

The doctor's visit is not built to pack in a layered interpretation of many weeks or months of raw data. In most practices, a 15-minute visit every 12 weeks is enough to make a decent decision about dosing amounts and to interpret some blood work. The continuous stream of data from patients' watches may be three months old by the time their doctor sees it. Patients want nearly real-time interpretation when they're trying to solve health problems. The more data they come across, the more problems they are bound to see.

Fitbit built a company on the premise that the device generating raw data was the product. They were wrong. Two other companies—Livongo and its acquirer, Teladoc—proved the point from opposite perspectives. Livongo built the story around the data and succeeded; and Teladoc dismantled it.

THE FITBIT BET

In 2014, Fitbit owned 68% of the U.S. fitness tracker market.[2] The company had solved one of the hardest problems in consumer electronics: getting people to wear something on their body all day, every day. Fitbit devices counted steps, tracked sleep, and monitored heart rate. In 2015, the company went public at a value above $6 billion. Shares peaked at $51.64.[3] The climb looked unstoppable. In November 2019, Google bought Fitbit for $2.1 billion. By that time, Fitbit's market share had collapsed to 4.1%.[4]

The usual story blames the competition. The Apple Watch ate the market, and Smartphone sensors made dedicated trackers feel redundant. That story isn't wrong, but it hides something more important. Fitbit had proof, from its own customers, that a different model worked, yet the company chose not to build it.

The Split

The proof came from corporate wellness programs. Seventy different Fortune 500 companies used Fitbit devices in employee health programs.[5] These programs wrapped the hardware in something the consumer market didn't have: goals, challenges, team competitions, coaching, and accountability. The Dayton Regional Transit Authority saved $2.3 million in employer healthcare costs over two years using Fitbit-based wellness programs.[6] John Hancock offered life insurance customers up to 15% off their premiums for wearing the device and hitting activity targets.[7] Across these corporate programs, documented healthcare savings averaged about $1,300 per participant per year, a 24.5% reduction in total costs.[8]

The consumer market told a different story. By early 2015, only half of Fitbit's 19 million registered users were still active, and *active* had a very low bar: the company counted anyone who logged 100 steps or opened the app once.[9] One out of three consumers stopped using the device within six months.[10] After a profitable 2015, Fitbit lost money every year. Total losses from 2016 through 2019 passed $887 million.[11]

The hardware was identical in both settings. The difference was whether the data was connected to interpretation. In corporate wellness, the device came wrapped in structure: step goals, leaderboards, coaches who actually checked in, and insurance discounts tied to activity. The structure told users what to do with the signal, and the corporate Fitbit produced $1,300 in annual health value per participant. In the consumer market, the same signal arrived with no structure. Users looked at the number, felt vaguely good or bad about it, and eventually put the device in a drawer.

Engagement Levels Are Not What Drives the Business

Fitbit's CEO, James Park, responded to concerns about falling user engagement with this: "Engagement levels aren't what drives the business."[12] He was technically right. Engagement didn't drive Fitbit's revenue; hardware sales did—but that was a choice they made. Whether a user wore the device for two years or two months, Fitbit captured about $87 per device purchase.[13] After the sale, whatever happened next was, from a revenue perspective, the user's problem. But if Fitbit captured $87 per device, and the employer captured about $1,300 per year in health savings, every dollar of that gap was attributable to the interpretation layer, or the storytelling. Fitbit could have been a wellness storytelling juggernaut if it had invested in behavioral infrastructure. It had the data systems, the user base, and the brand. It needed a subscription service on top of the hardware, priced to capture some fraction of the value the devices were already producing. As Park himself said, the company would "use technology to help people become healthier and more active . . . giving them data and inspiration and guidance."[14] Fitbit only built one of the three.

THE HARDWARE CHOICE

Hardware companies capture value at the moment of sale; subscription companies have to earn each month's renewal. Margins on wristbands are simple. Margins on coaching are complex. Fitbit was a hardware company. Becoming a coaching company would have meant becoming a different company. It wasn't irrational for them to stay in their lane.

Digital health platforms in obesity medicine have the Fitbit blind spot: their offers are weak on titration guidance, side-effect management, and helping patients set realistic expectations. This layer is what produces durable weight loss in patients and enduring long-term value on balance sheets. For about five years, these platforms took the simple margins, skipped the relationship, and let the employer, the insurer, or the patient figure out the rest.

Chapter 6 described Peloton making its version of the same mistake with bikes. Fitbit made it with wristbands. In both cases, the company that owned the customer also owned the data, but decided to monetize only the hardware. Peloton figured it out. Fitbit is still *very 2014.*

WHAT INTERPRETATION LOOKS LIKE

During Fitbit's rise, a company called Livongo launched with a different premise. They saw their hardware as a conduit to the real value of remaining connected to patients.

Livongo gave members with chronic conditions blood glucose meters, blood pressure cuffs, and scales. The devices uploaded readings automatically. When a glucose reading came back dangerously high or low, a Diabetes Response Specialist called the member within minutes. The specialist wasn't a physician. The role didn't require a medical degree. It required training in diabetes management, access to the member's data, and clear protocols for common situations. One specialist served several thousand members and averaged eight to nine member conversations per day.[15] This wasn't boutique medicine; it was a proactive intervention built to scale. Members also had access to health coaches 24 hours a day, who were available typically within 60 to 90 seconds of a patient reaching out.[16]

The model worked. Members averaged HbA1c reductions of 0.8 to 1.6 percentage points without changing medications. HbA1c is the three-month blood-sugar average that predicts long-term complications like kidney failure, nerve damage, diabetic eye disease, and heart attack.[17] Livongo documented $1,908 in yearly savings per diabetes member. Enrollment in employer programs reached 35% of the eligible population.[18] In 2019, Livongo went public at a $2.5 billion valuation.[19]

Livongo called its data science philosophy "AI+AI," an acronym for aggregate, interpret, apply, and iterate.[20] Livongo presented personalized signals directly to members, watched whether the recommendation changed behavior, and iterated when it didn't. Livongo built the infrastructure to do that work at scale, and the system learned from every interaction.

About 90% to 95% of Livongo's revenue came from monthly subscription fees rather than hardware sales.[21] The devices were the gateway to the relationship and its monetization. Livongo gave away the devices. The value was in the interpretation. The company was paid repeatedly because it delivered caring guidance over and over again. The rapid response call was the clinical intervention and the business model at the same time.

But the most important thing Livongo built wasn't the glucose tracking framework or the coaching platform. It was the alignment. Livongo's founders had diagnosed a structural problem that sits underneath most of healthcare's commercial failures. As Lee Shapiro, the company's CFO (Chief Financial Officer), put it, "if you're healthy, you're a lousy customer for most health systems because you don't come in for more visits, they can't do more procedures, they can't prescribe more tests. But if I take a lot longer to get healthy, I'm a revenue center."[22] The entire sick care model, the episodic model that requires disease to earn, was the thing Livongo set out to invert. And they did it with a simple structural choice: employers paid a flat monthly fee per member, but only for members who opted in and kept using the service. If a member disengaged, Livongo lost the revenue. If the member stayed healthy, the employer renewed. The incentives were aligned to improve patient health, which meant fewer sick days for employers and more employee productivity, which sustains net profit. "In some businesses, there's an inherent tension between who is paying you and who is using your products," said Chief Technology Officer Dave Engberg. "At Livongo, there was no conflict."[23]

That structural alignment between patient success and commercial success was the real product. Livongo was on its way to proving at scale that a healthcare company could grow by keeping people well rather than treating them when they got worse. Then the acquisition came. Livongo was absorbed into another company that still ran on the *more-visits-more-revenue* logic Livongo sought to replace.

The $18.5 Billion Acquisition

In August 2020, Teladoc Health announced it would buy Livongo for $18.5 billion.[24] The deal was framed as transformational. Teladoc was the dominant telehealth platform for on-demand physician visits in the United States, and Livongo brought the chronic care infrastructure Teladoc lacked. Together, they would cover more than 70 million lives and earn $1.3 billion in revenue. They ran a single platform that unified everything from acute visits to ongoing diabetes care around data and delivered it through digital channels,[25] thereby forming the first full-stack virtual care company. By February 2021, the combined market cap peaked above $45 billion.[26]

Eighteen months later, Teladoc was forced to write down $13.4 billion of the Livongo purchase. The company said the assets it had bought were worth a fraction of what it had paid.[27] The write-downs came in waves of $6.6 billion in the first quarter of 2022, $3.0 billion in the second quarter, and $3.8 billion in the fourth quarter; the full-year 2022 net loss reached $13.7 billion.[28] By late 2025, the stock traded around $7 per share, down 98% from its peak.[29] The market cap had collapsed from over $45 billion to approximately $1.3 billion.[30] Teladoc was worth less than what it had paid for Livongo alone.

The deal didn't fail because Livongo was failing. Livongo was profitable and growing, with documented clinical results. The $18.5 billion purchase price represented a $16 billion premium over the $2.5 billion valuation. This came from a real belief in the model's value. What Teladoc didn't understand was what produced that value.

In January 2023, Teladoc announced layoffs of 300 employees, or 6% of its non-clinician workforce. CEO Jason Gorevic pointed to *redundant roles born out of mergers* as a target.[31] Industry observers watched key Livongo staff leave in the months following the merger, and the institutional knowledge walked out the door with them.[32]

The Diabetes Response Specialist model shifted. In 2024 and 2025, the company began promoting *predictive AI modeling* and digital notifications as the way to keep members engaged.[33] The rapid response call shrank to a quiet push notification, replacing the human who had read the glucose spike, understood its context, and told the patient what to do in less than three minutes. The interpretation became optional. The patient could respond to the nudge or ignore it.

WHAT THE LIVONGO OUTCOME SHOWS

Pre-merger Livongo studies documented large HbA1c reductions, which justified employer adoption and investor confidence.[34] A 2024 report from the Peterson

Health Technology Institute analyzed Teladoc's diabetes offerings and found that HbA1c reductions ranged from 0.23 to 0.60 percentage points. Far lower than the Livongo days. Only three of the 10 studies reviewed met the threshold for clinical meaningfulness, which is a reduction of at least 0.5 percentage points.[35]

Glen Tullman, Livongo's founder, left shortly after the merger. By 2025, he was publicly critical of what had happened. The "after-the-fact-call-me-if-you-need-me model," he said, "has been proven time and time again to not improve outcomes."[36]

That is what Livongo had become. The company that proved human interpretation could scale had been converted by its acquirer into one that asked patients to make their own data mean something. Teladoc's leadership had understood the problem correctly: trained people who could read a glucose spike and call within minutes are expensive. But that mindset only looks at one side of the ledger. They tried to scale the Livongo model by diluting it, spreading resources thin, replacing specialists with automated alerts, and assuming the efficiency gains would offset the drop in effectiveness. The approach destroyed over $40 billion of value. By late 2025, visit-based fees made up over 50% of Teladoc's U.S. virtual care revenue, reflecting an accelerating shift away from the preventive subscription model.[37] The company drifted back toward the transactional urgent-care model it had set out to transcend.

Fitbit bet on a business model that lets someone else provide the interpretation layer and capture the ongoing value. Livongo combined data and interpretation into a single product, and it worked. Teladoc then scaled it back to sick care because they couldn't break out of the more-visits/more-revenue gambit. Obesity affects over 100 million Americans. Care delivered in one-to-one appointments won't work. But replacing it with superficial, synthetic notifications will fail too.

ENDNOTES

1. The Notorious B.I.G., *Mo Money Mo Problems*, Life After Death, Bad Boy Records, 1997.
2. Xiaoke Xu and Xin Wang, *Fitbit: The Business About Wrist*, no. W16264 (Ivey Publishing, Ivey Business School, Western University, 2016).
3. Xu and Wang, *Fitbit: The Business About Wrist*, 5.
4. "Google Is Buying Fitbit for $2.1 Billion, Betting on Fitness Wearables," Los Angeles Times, November 1, 2019, https://www.latimes.com/business/story/2019-11-01/google-to-buy-fitness-wearables-giant-fitbit-for-about-2-1-billion.
5. Regina E. Herzlinger et al., *Fitbit*, nos. 9-317–007 (Harvard Business School, 2021), 4.
6. Herzlinger et al., *Fitbit*, 7.
7. Xu and Wang, *Fitbit: The Business About Wrist*, 7.
8. "Fitbit Group Health Customers Demonstrate Corporate Wellness Programs Leads to Healthcare Savings," Google, October 4, 2016, https://blog.google/products/fitbit/fitbit-group-health-customers-demonstrate-corporate-wellness-programs-leads-healthcare-savings/.
9. Herzlinger et al., *Fitbit*, 2.
10. Xu and Wang, *Fitbit: The Business About Wrist*, 6.
11. Shamik Debnath et al., *Google: Targeting the Health Care Market with Fitbit*, no. W21356 (Ivey Publishing, Ivey Business School, Western University, 2021).
12. Herzlinger et al., *Fitbit*, 2.
13. Debnath et al., *Google: Targeting the Health Care Market with Fitbit*, 3.
14. Xu and Wang, *Fitbit: The Business About Wrist*, 6.
15. Adesh Surendra Jain et al., *The Teladoc and Livongo Merger*, SM-349 (Stanford Graduate School of Business, 2021), 6.
16. Ranjay Gulati et al., *Livongo: Scaling a Purpose-Driven Organization in Healthcare*, nos. 9-422–017 (Harvard Business School, 2021), 1.
17. Livongo Health Inc., *Return on Investment of the Livongo for Diabetes Program* (corporate white paper, 2021), 4; Jennifer B. Bollyky et al., "Remote Lifestyle Coaching Plus a Connected Glucose Meter with Certified Diabetes Educator Support Improves Glucose and Weight Loss for People with Type 2 Diabetes," *Journal of Diabetes Research* 2018 (May 2018): 3961730, https://doi.org/10.1155/2018/3961730; Janelle Downing et al., "Use of a Connected Glucose Meter and Certified Diabetes Educator Coaching to Decrease the Likelihood of Abnormal Blood Glucose Excursions: The Livongo for Diabetes Program," *Journal of Medical Internet Research* 19, no. 7 (2017): e234, https://doi.org/10.2196/jmir.6659.
18. Jain et al., *The Teladoc and Livongo Merger*, 7.
19. Jain et al., *The Teladoc and Livongo Merger*, 7; Livongo Health Inc., *Form S-1 Registration Statement* (U.S. Securities and Exchange Commission EDGAR, 2019), https://www.sec.gov/Archives/edgar/data/1639225/000119312519185159/d731249ds1.htm.

20. Ranjay Gulati et al., *Livongo: Scaling a Purpose-Driven Organization in Healthcare,* n.d., 8.
21. Jain et al., *The Teladoc and Livongo Merger*, 7; Livongo Health Inc., *Form S-1 Registration Statement.*
22. Gulati et al., *Livongo: Scaling a Purpose-Driven Organization in Healthcare*, 4.
23. Ibid.
24. "Teladoc Health and Livongo Merge to Create New Standard in Global Healthcare Delivery, Access and Experience," news release, Teladoc Health, August 5, 2020, https://ir.teladochealth.com/news-and-events/investor-news/press-release-details/2020/Teladoc-Health-and-Livongo-Merge-to-Create-New-Standard-in-Global-Healthcare-Delivery-Access-and-Experience/default.aspx.
25. Jain et al., *The Teladoc and Livongo Merger*, 1.
26. Jon Quast, "Here's Why Teladoc Health Stock Fell 16% in February," The Motley Fool, March 4, 2021, https://www.fool.com/investing/2021/03/04/heres-why-teladoc-health-stock-fell-16-in-february/.
27. LIVE NATION ENTERTAINMENT, INC., *Form 10-K for the Fiscal Year Ended December 30, 2024*, Form 10-K (Washington, DC, 2024), https://www.sec.gov/Archives/edgar/data/1335258/000133525825000028/lyv-20241231.htm#id16a83bb3b7a48f59c925134d5705b64_61; Heather Landi, "Teladoc Sinks $13.7B Loss in 2022 Tied to Livongo Acquisition," FIERCE Healthcare, February 23, 2023, https://www.fiercehealthcare.com/health-tech/teladoc-sinks-137b-loss-2022-tied-plummeting-value-livongo-acquisition?utm.
28. "Teladoc Health, Inc.—Financial Info—SEC Filings," 2022, https://ir.teladoc.com/financial-info/sec-filings/default.aspx; Rebecca Pifer, "Teladoc Reports Historic Net Loss of $13.7B in 2022," Healthcare Dive, February 23, 2023, https://www.healthcaredive.com/news/teladoc-historic-net-loss-137b-2022/643213/.
29. "Teladoc Health—11 Year Stock Price History," Macrotrends, accessed January 2, 2026, https://www.macrotrends.net/stocks/charts/TDOC/teladoc-health/stock-price-history.
30. "Teladoc Health Market Cap 2014–2025," Macrotrends, accessed January 6, 2026, https://www.macrotrends.net/stocks/charts/TDOC/teladoc-health/market-cap.
31. Emily Olson, "Teladoc Health Lays off 300 Employees to Cut Costs," Mobi Health News, January 18, 2023, https://www.mobihealthnews.com/news/teladoc-health-lays-300-employees-cut-costs; Annie Burky, "Teladoc Lets Go 300 Employees, 6% of Its Non-Clinician Workforce," FIERCE Healthcare, January 18, 2023, https://www.fiercehealthcare.com/telehealth/teladoc-health-announced-email-employees-it-would-be-laying-300-employees-6-its-non.
32. Gulati et al., *Livongo: Scaling a Purpose-Driven Organization in Healthcare,* 16; Arundhati Parmar, "With Livongo, Did Zane Burke Sell a Lemon to Teladoc's Jason Gorevic?," *MedCity News*, January 30, 2023, https://medcitynews.com/2023/01/with-livongo-did-zane-burke-sell-a-lemon-to-teladocs-jason-gorevic/.

33. "Teladoc Health's Predictive AI-Modeling Leads to Increased Engagement Among Diabetes Members, Driving Additional A1c Reduction, New Research Shows," Teladoc Health, June 24, 2024, https://www.teladochealth.com/newsroom/press/Teladoc-Healths-predictive-AI-modeling-leads-to-increased-engagement-among-diabetes-members-driving-additional-A1c-reduction-new-research-shows.
34. Livongo Health Inc., *Return on Investment of the Livongo for Diabetes Program*, 4; Bollyky et al., "Remote Lifestyle Coaching Plus a Connected Glucose Meter with Certified Diabetes Educator Support Improves Glucose and Weight Loss for People with Type 2 Diabetes."
35. *Digital Diabetes Management Solutions: Health Technology Assessment*, Health Technology Assessment (Peterson Health Technology Institute, 2024), https://phti.org/wp-content/uploads/sites/3/2024/03/PHTI-Digital-Diabetes-Mgmt-Assessment-Report-v1.0.pdf.
36. Arundhati Parmar, "Is Glen Tullman a Hypocrite or a Victim of the System He Aimed to Disrupt?," *MedCity News*, February 13, 2025, https://medcitynews.com/2025/02/is-glen-tullman-a-hypocrite-or-a-victim-of-the-system-he-aimed-to-disrupt/.
37. Teladoc Health, "Teladoc Health Reports Fourth Quarter and Full Year 2025 Results," accessed May 9, 2026, https://ir.teladochealth.com/news-and-events/investor-news/press-release-details/2026/Teladoc-Health-Reports-Fourth-Quarter-and-Full-Year-2025-Results/default.aspx.

CHAPTER 8

ZARA IS BUILT TO LISTEN

On a Tuesday afternoon in Milan, a woman in her mid-thirties stands in front of a display table stacked with folded sweaters. She picks up a navy crewneck, holds it against her chest, and sets it down. She moves to the burgundy version two feet away, lifts it, examines the fabric, and puts it back. Back to the navy. This time she unfolds it completely, checks the size tag, refolds it carefully, and places it back on the stack. She does not leave. She circles the table once, picks up the navy sweater again, and walks toward the fitting rooms before stopping halfway, turning back, and setting it down a third time. Then she leaves the store empty-handed.

Elena, the store manager, watches from near the register. She has seen this exact sequence four times today with four different customers and involving the same navy sweater. Elena pulls out her handheld device and types a short note: navy crewneck, high try-on rate, low conversion, customers hesitating at price point or fit.[1] The observation takes less than a minute to record.

Elena is watching customers the way a clinician watches a patient in an exam room. Not just listening to what they say, but noticing what they do when they think no one is paying attention. The hesitation. The return to the same item. The moment when interest turns into doubt. This is where listening begins, before any technology, before any data system. It begins with a person who has learned to notice.

By Wednesday morning, Elena's note will arrive at Zara's headquarters in Arteixo, Spain, in the Galicia region, where reports from over 2,000 stores in 96 countries flow in every single day.[2] The building that receives these reports belongs to Inditex, Zara's parent company. The reports contain unit sales by SKU, by hour, and by store. They list return rates by item and stock flow metrics. The point-of-sale computers capture and move all of this data in real time to Arteixo.[3]

But the numbers only tell half the story. Elena's observation about the woman with the navy sweater is the other half. Store managers carry those handheld devices to record what the sales data cannot see. The discarded sweater SKUs in Elena's store alone are one thing. But the same note from Barcelona, Brussels, and Berlin is a pattern.[4]

Typically, demand for specific medications is recorded in fragmented streams across thousands of independent practices, hundreds of pharmacy systems, and dozens of insurance databases. The digital health platforms with GLP-1 prescription programs have each written millions of prescriptions over the last few years. They can listen to patients in ways the traditional medical system cannot because the data is in one place. A patient in Ohio who struggles with nausea in week three could be one of thousands. A patient in Arizona who stops responding to messages after the second dose increase could be a canary in the coal mine for what we know is a low-retention system. These are not isolated events. They are patterns in need of a systematic supportive response.

HOW INFORMATION MOVES

Every morning, Zara's store managers check their handheld devices to see which new designs are open for ordering.[5] They review what sold yesterday in their own store and in nearby stores like theirs. They place orders twice a week from a constantly updating list.

Zara's fashion is famously fast, but so is the speed of its information handling. Zara's design team works in one open space at headquarters.[6] They sit near the buyers and merchandisers who read store feedback. They, in turn, sit near the planners who schedule production. Physical proximity means a conversation can happen in minutes. In most companies, the same exchange would take days of email and Slack messages winding through three departments.

Zara has no chief designer.[7] Most fashion companies place creative power in the hands of one person whose vision defines the brand. Zara spreads creative power across 350 designers, each one empowered to approve products based on data. The flat structure reaches beyond design. There are few formal meetings and committees. Information flows through conversations and shared workspaces, not through long chains of approval.[8]

The founder, Amancio Ortega, never had an office. He worked in an open space in the design area, close to the teams around him.[9] His daughter Marta Ortega, who became chair in 2022,[10] does not have an office either. This was not just about speed. It was about keeping the subject matter experts embedded in daily decision making. Ortega understood that the cost of expertise—350 designers, buyers who travel constantly, and highly skilled store managers trained to observe—was not a waste. It was the mechanism that prevented far more expensive failures downstream. Empowered expertise lowers design failure rates, customer acquisition cost, and improves brand loyalty. Ortega saw this was true of luxury brands and brought it across Europe and the world. When you listen with real expertise and respond to what you hear, you build things people actually want.

Glen Tullman made the same structural choice when he built Livongo. He filled leadership with doctors who had experience in managing their own chronic diseases. They were not decorative; they were embedded in product decisions, in care protocols, and in how the company listened to members.[11] Both Ortega and Tullman understood that people gravitate toward systems built by people who genuinely understand what they need—Ortega in the design space and doctors inside Livongo. Experts are only expensive if they are not empowered and embedded. The large digital medicine platforms today are not paying attention to this lesson. They optimize for operational efficiency and overlook the fact that well-deployed expertise creates compounding loyalty.

Designers receive daily sales data, daily customer feedback, and daily trend reports. When stores report that customers want a red version of a successful blue jacket, designers can sketch the new color that afternoon. If the fabric is already in inventory, and Zara keeps basic fabrics on hand for exactly this reason, production can begin within days.[12]

The 350 designers create 18,000 new product designs per year.[13] They can do this because the listening system tells them what to design. They are not guessing nor responding to the whims of the C-suite. They are responding to real customer requests pulled from 2,000 stores. The system gives each designer leverage: each one is far more productive because they know what will sell before they sketch it.

Amancio Ortega understood that being inside the system, close to the people making decisions, was what made it all work. Tullman understood the same thing. Both knew that listening at scale and hearing the real needs of the people you serve requires proximity. Not just physical proximity—though that matters—but structural proximity. In other words, being close enough to the work that you can hear what is actually happening.

In obesity medicine, expert clinicians are scarce. But a *listening* infrastructure transforms how clinicians spend their time. I have spent years building and working both brick-and-mortar and digital obesity medicine practices. I have read and responded to thousands of patient messages about weight loss.

When patients send messages because they are enraged about their slow progress, they are not actually angry; they are terrified. They are worried they are among the small group of nonresponders. They carry the weight of every failed diet, and every time, they blame themselves for not having enough willpower. They are caught in a self-deprecating failure loop. What they need to know is that they are not alone. They need to be treated gently. I came to this realization because of the patterns that emerged over years of listening.

When a patient asks for a significant change in their dose or wants to switch medications, they are often trying to address a budget issue. They are often too embarrassed to say "my insurance won't cover this" or "I can't afford that." Many patients hesitate to ask their doctors to make changes to the plan because they fear appearing needy or ignorant. Usually, if they have asked for a change, they have not done so lightly. My job is to acknowledge that these medications are expensive, and to deploy coverage and cost mechanisms to help them figure it out.

Elena noticed the customer's hesitation in her body language—the return to the same sweater and the moment when interest turned into doubt. Clinicians notice the same things. When we are empowered to act on what we see, we can respond in ways that acknowledge the patient's true needs. In this, we build trust. And trust is everything.

RESPONDING TO PATIENT NEEDS

Three decisions enable Zara's response time. Each one involved accepting a cost that most competitors refused to pay. The first is where manufacturing happens. Most fashion companies send 100% of production to Asia to keep labor costs low. Zara makes more than half of its fashion items in Spain, Portugal, Turkey, and Morocco. These are higher-wage places, but they are close to headquarters and dramatically cut lead times.[14] It also diversifies the supply chains to protect against major shocks. The stages that matter most, design and cutting, happen in factories near the design team. A new design can move from sketch to a European store shelf in two weeks. Inditex accepted higher labor costs in exchange for flexibility and speed.[15]

Second, Zara reserves 85% of its factory capacity for in-season adjustments.[16] Traditional manufacturing treats unused capacity as a problem to be eliminated. Zara treats it as the very thing that makes responsiveness possible.

Over 50% of Zara's clothes are designed and made mid-season, after the company has real sales data instead of forecasts.[17] The opening collection is a hypothesis. Customer response tells the company which guesses were right and which need to change. Reserve capacity allows change to happen in weeks rather than months.

I find this idea clinically intuitive. In my practice, I do not ask a patient to commit to an entire treatment plan on day one and then refuse to adjust it. The initial prescription is a hypothesis. The patient's response tells me what to change. But most obesity medicine programs lack the structural capacity to respond to what they learn. They prescribe according to rigid protocols and cannot adapt when a patient says they need something different.

The third decision is that all Zara garments pass through one of two highly automated distribution centers in Spain.[18] Clothes arrive already tagged and priced, ready for sale the moment they reach stores. The distribution center can sort and ship an order within eight hours. A shipment leaving Arteixo arrives at a European store within 24 to 48 hours. The centralization looks inefficient on paper, but centralized shipping means headquarters can see the entire global inventory in real time and send stock to where demand shows up. A style selling faster than expected in Germany can pull inventory that is moving slowly in France, within the same shipment cycle.

THE ZARA CULTURE

Zara does not give up localization with this centralization. They do both well. Store managers act like entrepreneurs. Each one has the authority to order what they think will sell in their specific neighborhood.[19] They place orders twice a week based on their read of local customers. Two stores in the same city can end up with different inventory by the end of a season. Different patient populations need different configurations of care. A 28-year-old tech worker in San Francisco has different barriers to medication adherence than a 62-year-old retiree in rural Ohio. Scale and personalization are not at odds if the system functions well.

Personalization is only possible because customers care about Zara. They come back even if they left empty-handed on their last trip. They spend time trying on clothes in the store. They have opinions about what they want. The listening infrastructure has something real and organic to listen to. Customers feel something about the brand. That feeling is not manufactured through marketing or incentivized testimonials. It comes from the experience of being heard and seeing the system respond. The navy skirt appears because someone asked for it. The sleeves got shorter because customers said they were too long. These are not loyalty points or email campaigns. It is the accumulated experience of mattering.

Livongo insisted on capitalizing their word for customers—*Members*. Not patients; *Members*. They belonged to something.[20] They trusted Livongo, and Livongo earned that trust. The relationship was not transactional.

I have built clinical protocols for three large platforms in the obesity medicine space. I have always fought to connect the clinician more closely with the patient. I built systems to warmly welcome every new patient with a simple, sincere message about their assessment. It shows up in reviews. It matters to them that within these monolithic platforms, a real, caring human is overseeing a difficult time in their lives. Belonging cannot be manufactured. It cannot be bought. It has to be real. Customers and patients feel this so deeply.

Digital health platforms competing for market share have designed their systems for transactions. Wallet shares can never emerge from there because patients don't matter—their payments do. Patients have no issue switching between platforms that do not hear them because they have nothing to lose. The listening infrastructure can be technically perfect and the response time can be measured in minutes, but if the patient does not feel that someone inside the system genuinely cares whether they succeed, they will leave the moment a cheaper option appears. That is the difference between market share and wallet share. In 2026, that difference is everything.

ZARA'S LISTEN-RESPOND LOOP

Listening is everyone's job at Zara. New employees spend time learning to observe customers, regardless of their formal role.[21] The culture expects that listening and responding are part of every position. Elena's reports from her store are collated with the reports from stores across Europe.

The analyst walks over to the design area, which is close by, and mentions the pattern to a designer. The designer pulls up the original sketch and considers Elena's note about how the sweater fits. The designer makes a few adjustments based on recent well-reviewed sweaters and sends the new pattern to the cutting facility.[22] Automatic cutting machines cut the navy fabric. A small batch of updated sweaters is sewn within a few days, and the finished garments are shipped to the distribution center. They are sorted, tagged, and shipped to trial stores, including Elena's. She is empowered by the fact that her expertise matters and is motivated to keep listening and observing.[23] Zara's superpower is to *continuously sense what customers want to buy and then respond* on the fly.[24]

The loop is continuous because the more you listen and respond, the richer the insights. Insights beget more of the same as the loyalty deepens and wallet share emerges. Zara's loops are what Livongo called "AI+AI": *aggregate, interpret + apply, iterate.*[25] Livongo aggregated glucose readings and patient messages, applied the expert interpretation layer, and responded promptly. They intervened with a phone call, a coaching session, and/or a suggestion for food. And they iterated by watching whether the intervention worked and adjusting if it did not. Each complete loop generates learning. Livongo did this for each member but this same loop also inspired their next product offerings. Zara's version runs through fabrics and storefronts; Livongo's runs through blood sugar readings and health coaches.

After decades of systematic listening and responding, Zara's prediction accuracy is remarkable. The company reports a 1% design failure rate versus about 10% across the industry.[26] The advantage comes from a commitment to listening and years of teaching the system which signals matter.

The markdown data tells the same story. Zara discounts about 15% of its items, while the fashion industry as a whole usually marks down around 50% of its inventory.[27] Customers visit Zara stores in Spain an average of 17 times a year. They visit competitors an average of three times a year.[28] Because new items arrive constantly—twice-weekly replenishment versus the seasonal refreshes of competitors—customers come back often to see what is new. Each visit is a chance to sell and a chance to watch. Each observation feeds the loop.

Zara's two-week design-to-shelf cycle is not only about speed. It is about closing the loop while the signal is still valid. The woman who wanted the navy sweater will come back soon. She will see the updated fit and try it on. Elena will watch and learn there, too.

A quick response to a patient's question is not just about their satisfaction; it is about closing the loop while they are still engaged. If they report nausea, they get a simple management strategy right away. The system watches whether the nausea score improves and whether the patient keeps taking the medication. This is the infrastructure that most patients on GLP-1s lack. Each complete loop refines which interventions work for which patients.

This is why a listen-respond system is hard to replicate. A competitor can buy the same handheld devices Zara uses. But without a commitment to listening that assigns meaning to the signals, the devices are just expensive ways to send messages. What creates advantage is the accumulated learning from continuous response loops. Year-one prediction accuracy enables leverage in year two, which enables scale in year three, which enables better prediction in year four. And all of it builds wallet share, which funds patient success infrastructure instead of more internet ads.

ENDNOTES

1. Andrew McAfee et al., *Zara: IT for Fast Fashion*, nos. 9-604–081 (Harvard Business School, 2007), 5–6.
2. Antonio Moreno, *Zara: An Integrated Store and Online Model (A)*, nos. 9-620–073 (Harvard Business School, 2021).
3. Vanessa Burbano et al., *Zara's Sustainability Dilemma*, no. 190401 (Columbia Business School, 2022), 2; McAfee et al., *Zara: IT for Fast Fashion*, 2.
4. McAfee et al., *Zara: IT for Fast Fashion*, 3–4; Guillerma D'Andrea and David Arnold, *Zara*, nos. 9-503–050 (Harvard Business School, 2003), 4.
5. McAfee et al., *Zara: IT for Fast Fashion*, 5–6.
6. Destination Innovation, *Innovation Lessons from Fashion Leader, Zara*, Innovation Examples & Lessons, April 29, 2012, https://www.destination-innovation.com/innovation-lessons-from-fashion-leader-zara/; Martin Roll, "The Secret of Zara's Success: A Culture of Customer Co-Creation," *Martin Roll*, November 7, 2021, https://martinroll.com/resources/articles/strategy/the-secret-of-zaras-success-a-culture-of-customer-co-creation/.
7. Martin Roll, "The Secret of Zara's Success."
8. McAfee et al., *Zara: IT for Fast Fashion*, 3–4.
9. Martin Roll, "The Secret of Zara's Success."
10. "The Board of Directors of Inditex Agrees to Appoint Marta Ortega as Chairwoman, and Óscar García Maceiras as Chief Executive Officer," INDITEX, November 30, 2021, https://www.inditex.com/itxcomweb/us/en/press/news-detail/82af130d-3711-4a68-99ca-6e56113083e2/the-board-of-directors-of-inditex-agrees-to-appoint-marta-ortega-as-chairwoman-and-scar-garca-maceiras-as-chief-executive-officer.
11. Ranjay Gulati et al., *Livongo: Scaling a Purpose-Driven Organization in Healthcare*, nos. 9-422–017 (Harvard Business School, 2021).
12. Pnina Feldman et al., *Can Zara Fast-Forward Fashion?*, no. UV9154 (University of Virginia Darden Business Publishing, 2021), 4–5; McAfee et al., *Zara: IT for Fast Fashion*, 3–4.
13. Destination Innovation, *Innovation Lessons from Fashion Leader, Zara.*
14. Feldman et al., *Can Zara Fast-Forward Fashion?*, 4; Burbano et al., *Zara's Sustainability Dilemma*, 3.
15. Ibid.
16. Feldman et al., *Can Zara Fast-Forward Fashion?*, 4.
17. Feldman et al., *Can Zara Fast-Forward Fashion?*, 4; D'Andrea and Arnold, *Zara*, 4.
18. D'Andrea and Arnold, *Zara*, 4.
19. McAfee et al., *Zara: IT for Fast Fashion*, 3, 5–6; Feldman et al., *Can Zara Fast-Forward Fashion?*, 5.
20. Gulati et al., *Livongo: Scaling a Purpose-Driven Organization in Healthcare.*
21. Martin Roll, "The Secret of Zara's Success."
22. D'Andrea and Arnold, *Zara*, 4.

23. Ibid.
24. McAfee et al., *Zara: IT for Fast Fashion*, 7.
25. Gulati et al., *Livongo: Scaling a Purpose-Driven Organization in Healthcare.*
26. D'Andrea and Arnold, *Zara*, 3.
27. Burbano et al., *Zara's Sustainability Dilemma*, 4; Feldman et al., *Can Zara Fast-Forward Fashion?*; Dan Doiron, *Zara: The Evolving Fast-Fashion Industry*, no. W34418 (Ivey Publishing, Ivey Business School, Western University, 2023).
28. Doiron, *Zara: The Evolving Fast-Fashion Industry*, 3.

Part III

The Canopy: Building the Infrastructure for Patient Success

CHAPTER 9

THE TWO LAST MILES

On a Tuesday in July, Marcus pulls his refrigerated van into the parking lot of a small apartment complex in suburban Columbus at 2:47 PM. The complex has eight units, is two stories, and has vinyl siding. This is it. He is 17 minutes behind schedule. The packages in the back contain expensive and essential medications, including semaglutide and tirzepatide. The radio-frequency identification tag shows that the cargo has remained at 36°F for the past six hours. He has two hours before the cooling packs expire, and cold chain shipping is at risk.

Marcus looks for apartment 4C. There is no buzzer label for apartment 4C. He tries the building super. No answer. He tries adjacent apartments. A woman's voice comes through the intercom: "I don't know who lives in 4C." He calls the phone number and gets voicemail. He leaves a message. The medication that traveled 800 miles in 48 hours just failed in the final hundred yards.

This is the *last-mile problem*: the disproportionate difficulty and cost of completing the final leg of delivery to an individual consumer. Everything upstream can be optimized with automated sorting, climate-controlled warehouses and routing algorithms that sequence 200 stops per driver. The last mile remains stubbornly particular. A missing buzzer label, congested traffic, or a recipient not at home can make the last mile an agonizing crawl.

Last-mile delivery costs were 53% of total shipping costs as of 2024, up from 41% in 2018.[1] The term originated in 1980s telecommunications, describing the technical and economic difficulty of connecting individual end users to the primary network.[2] Trunk lines could spread costs across thousands of subscribers. The final connection served one customer, and the infrastructure could only be amortized over that single customer. This created an economic bottleneck that has since migrated into every consumer-facing logistics industry.

Supply chain managers built a discipline around solving it. They orient around the *Seven Rights*: right product, right customer, right quantity, right condition, right place, right time, right cost. Miss one, and the order has failed.[3] The *Perfect Order Index* turns that principle into a score. It evaluates each shipment on four operational dimensions: delivered on time, complete, damage-free, and accurately documented. A company that hits 99% on each of the four dimensions still scores only 96% overall (0.99 × 0.99 × 0.99 × 0.99). Drop each dimension to 90%, and the index crashes to 65.6%. The calculation is multiplicative, not averaged, because the customer's experience is binary: it was good enough, or it was not. An order that arrives on time and is complete but damaged is not 75% successful.[4]

Businesses that sell obesity medications are rapidly solving this *physical* last mile. Telehealth platforms help with streamlining the prescription process. Vertically integrated pharmacies manage dispensing. Cold chain logistics preserve medication integrity in transit. Digital health platforms generate billions of dollars in revenue annually through subscription models built on optimized home delivery.[5]

In the United States, patients can order these medications just like they order groceries. Thanks to supply chain science, there is a beautifully efficient delivery system for the most powerful obesity drugs in history. And patients still, for the most part, stop taking them within a year.[6]

This is the *second* last mile and the second moment of truth. The physical last mile ends when the box reaches the patient's hands. The *clinical* last mile begins in that same moment and runs for years. Every upstream investment in obesity medicine—the billions in research and development, the manufacturing scale-up, the distribution networks, and the coverage negotiations—either converts to value or evaporates in the years following the medication's arrival. The generational breakthroughs in obesity medication succeed or fail based on whether any given patient, in any given circumstance, can stay on treatment long enough to realize its long-term benefits.

This is why this physician is writing a business book. Someone who lives every day in the second last mile needs to say it clearly enough that the people making upstream decisions can hear it. Digital health companies in this market are not selling medications. They are selling enduring well-being and health transformation to millions of people, each with different goals and needs.

The physical last mile has a measurement discipline, a playbook, and 70 years of operational research behind it. The clinical last mile has none of these that are actually set for the future. No supply chain framework captures what happens after the box is opened, because what happens next is not logistics. It is human behavior, clinical complexity, and the slow work of sustainable change.

THE MONOCROP

Part II of this book examined companies to highlight an important aspect of the obesity market today. Apple showed that transaction-optimized pricing cannibalizes relationship-optimized pricing. Ticketmaster showed that artificial scarcity trains customers to seek alternatives that the company cannot control. Peloton showed that hardware and content are not the product; the instructor relationship and the community are. Fitbit showed that uninterpreted data is noise that customers cannot act on. Zara showed that a listening infrastructure—the operational capacity to detect what is happening in the field and respond quickly—is a competitive moat.

Each case study is a look back at what I call a *monocrop* business problem that was resolved with an ecosystem solution. In agriculture, the farmer who plants only one crop and optimizes everything for that crop may have a high return for a few harvests in a row. But monocrops are fragile. They are brittle in the face of system shocks, depend on constant external inputs, and succeed through extraction. They are in constant tension with nature. Integration, diversification, and the welcoming of organized complexity are what make a successful ecosystem, in farming and in business.

The prevailing digital health model in obesity medicine is a monocrop. The crop is the prescription. The expensive fertilizer is the acquisition cost. The harvest is whatever revenue can be extracted before the patient leaves. There is no ecosystem underneath, or what I call transformation infrastructure. When the price drops, when the competitor enters, when the patient stalls early and decides this isn't working, the system will not hold.

> ***"A forest is much more than what you see."***
> ***—Suzanne Simard***

The alternative is not a better monocrop. It is a different kind of system entirely.

THE CANOPY FRAMEWORK

Imagine a forest canopy instead. Multiple species at multiple heights, each occupying a niche that the others cannot fill, each strengthening the others by being there. Complex root systems, many species of trees and their rising trunks extending to diverse and interconnected crowns in the canopy where they are seen and fed by the sun. Underneath it all, an invisible network of fungal threads, the mycorrhizal layer, that connects the trees and lets the forest function as one organism rather than as a collection of individuals competing for the same patch of ground.

This is the Canopy (see Figure 9.1). It is the name for what transformation infrastructure looks like when built as an ecosystem rather than a linear supply chain with sequential nodes. Human beings do not work like this. Like forests, our connections are nonlinear and reciprocal, and the space between us is uneven.

The seven components represent the trunks in the Canopy. Each is a column of infrastructure that carries part of what the patient will eventually experience, presented to them at the crown:

The Canopy held up by seven trunks, fed by one soil, made living by what passes between.

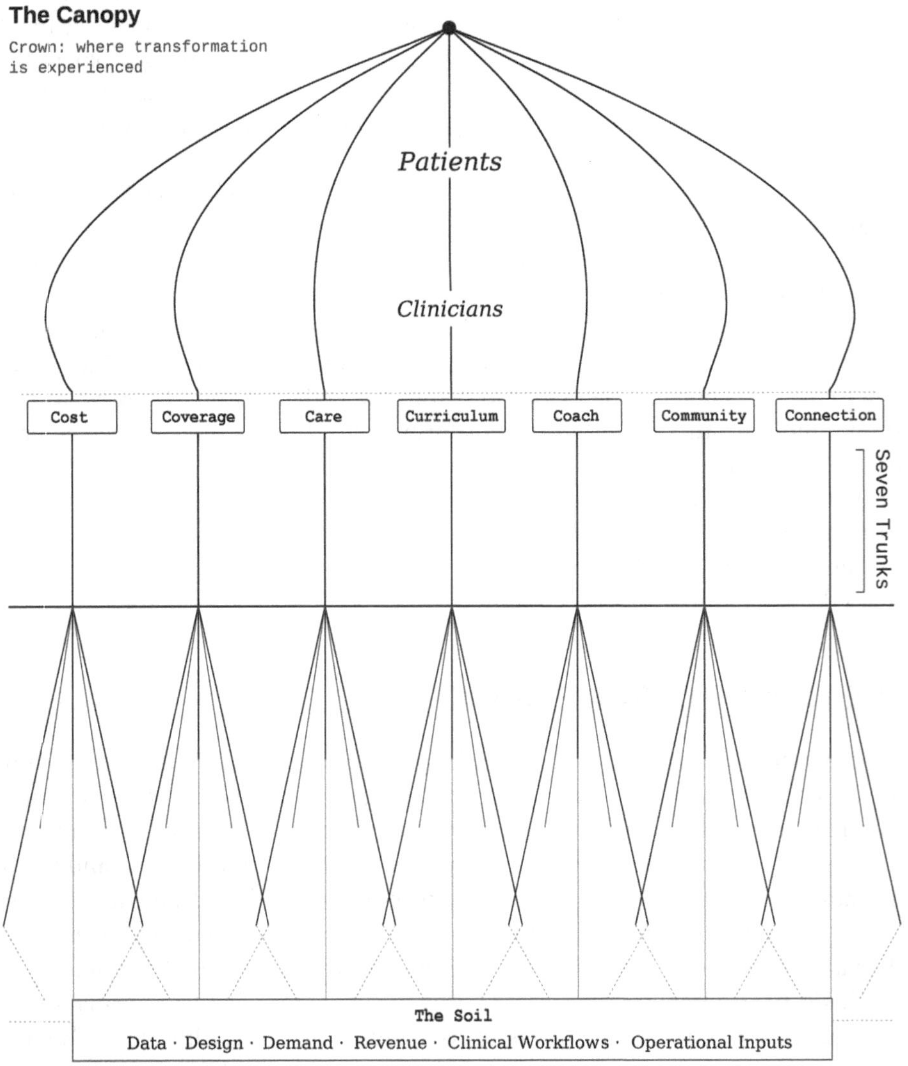

Figure 9.1 The Canopy Framework.

1. *Cost* is the pricing architecture that enables the program to exist inside a sustainable economic model
2. *Coverage* is the access infrastructure, insurance, employer partnerships, and bridge protocols—everything that gets a patient to treatment in the first place
3. *Care* is where clinical judgment resides: prescribing, titration, and the matching of clinical intensity to patient complexity
4. *Curriculum* is what the patient needs to know about the disease, the medication, and the predictable arc of treatment in order to succeed in the long term
5. *Coach* is the human and AI-augmented relationship that helps the patient act on what they know
6. *Community* is the peer infrastructure that tells them they are not alone and not broken
7. *Connection* is the listening infrastructure that detects when something is going wrong before the patient says so and ensures that the platform's relationship with the patient is not defined by discrete episodes of care but by a continuous experience of growth and healing

The root system is what feeds the trunks. It is data, design, consumer demand, revenue, clinical workflows, operational inputs, and every resource that flows into the components to strengthen them.

Within the Canopy itself, the patient experiences transformation. Patients do not see that one trunk is Cost and another is Care. They experience the components as a single, immersive ecosystem that feeds them, shades them, and changes the conditions in which they try to grow. It is the emergent layer, visible from below, produced by every trunk together.

A healthy forest is self-fulfilling. Sun and rain nourish the soil, the soil feeds the roots, the roots strengthen the trunks, and the trunks hold up the canopy. A healthy canopy produces the conditions for the next cycle. A transformed patient shares their experience, bringing more patients into the flywheel of growth. This strengthens the Canopy while lowering the costs of acquisition. A transformed patient remains loyal to the Canopy even after their hardest moments, allowing both to live off the momentum of earlier success and wisdom gained without raising the cost of treatment.

The mycorrhizal layer is the connective tissue that enables the system to share resources between its components. Simard's research at the University of British Columbia has shown that the fungal threads beneath a real forest move nutrients and warning signals between trees, allowing the forest to function as one organism.[7] It is the data flowing between the components, the shared patient record, and the listen-respond loops. The components are not seven services running in parallel. They are an ecosystem held together by what passes between them in the roots, soil, and the Canopy.

A program can have all seven components for transformation and still fail to create it. The integration of components throughout the forest is what distinguishes colocated services from an integrated system. Without designing for a complete system, you end up with an expensive monocrop. Monocrops are easy to measure, and ecosystems are not.

RETENTION DOES NOT MATTER

Retention is the wrong target. It is a trailing indicator of something else, and if you optimize for it directly, you end up building the same monoculture in nicer packaging. A patient can be retained by inertia, by a difficult cancellation flow, or by the absence of an alternative. I believe this explains the early success of the first digital health companies to sell obesity medications online.

The real target is transformation. A patient who understands their condition, accepts the current standard of long-term treatment for a lifelong disease, manages their dosing, adapts their diet, and navigates side effects is a transformed patient. Retention follows transformation, the way a robust harvest follows a healthy ecosystem.

This is also why a digital health platform cannot use the same measurement system as a grocery delivery service to decide if it is succeeding. Fast shipping and good online forms are the basic cost of entry in scaled obesity medicine platforms. What matters are the indicators of transformation—of an emerging Canopy.

THE CANOPY FRAMEWORK KEY PERFORMANCE INDICATORS

How do you know if you are actually helping a patient change? When I started writing this book, I realized that we have no system for measuring this work in digital health. Every business metric available is designed for the physical last mile, the one that gets the medication to the human. None of them measure the clinical last mile, which is getting the human to choose to take their medication as part of their health plan each and every month.

What if all of this scientific advancement—some of the most historic applications of modern biochemistry, immunology, and neuroscience—fails because we did not build in what we know about humans? We are notoriously irrational. We tend to underestimate long-term gains and overestimate short-term costs, and we block our own movement in a healthier direction when we do not understand why it matters.

This entire book asserts that the way to succeed in obesity medicine is to build a space where patients can change on their own terms. That means creating a system for transformation and figuring out how to design it for use across delivery models as different as a fully digital platform, a brick-and-mortar clinic, and a hybrid program—with or without AI-augmentation. It means tracking patients' behavior while in the system so that you can capture the change as it crescendos into transformation. And it means ensuring the change produces meaningful patient outcomes. The entire Canopy framework is designed to ensure that whatever you are building actually matches the lived experience of people with obesity. That is the entire job.

In Part III, I will share a practical definition of each of the seven components and explore why they matter. I will also share key performance indicators (KPIs) to measure the success of that component and its contribution to the success of the system—the Canopy itself. This is how a company can know that it is solving the clinical last mile. Indicators of transformation show up in what patients do inside the program, its design process, and the actual changes to patients' lives as a result of the program:

- *Patient behavior KPIs* measure what patients do that they would not otherwise do. They are the things you can point to and say, "This person *uses* the product." Not simply, "This person *likes* the product" or, "This person *reports satisfaction* with the product." This person reorders, escalates, returns, engages, and refers.
- *Program stewardship KPIs* measure what the program does to make that behavior possible. Stewardship is the operational expression of intent, the response time, the workflow completeness, and the structural readiness to deliver each component.
- *Outcome KPIs* measure what changes in the patient's body and life as a result. These are anchored to the International Consortium for Health Outcomes Measurement (ICHOM) Adult Obesity Standard Set, the set of outcomes that an international consensus of clinicians and patients agreed are the ones worth measuring in adult obesity care.[8] The convergence between what a practicing clinician sees in the room and what the ICHOM panel validates through formal consensus gives the framework its clinical authority.
- *Whole Canopy KPIs* measure whether the whole ecosystem is producing the transformation that no single component could produce alone (see Figure 9.2).

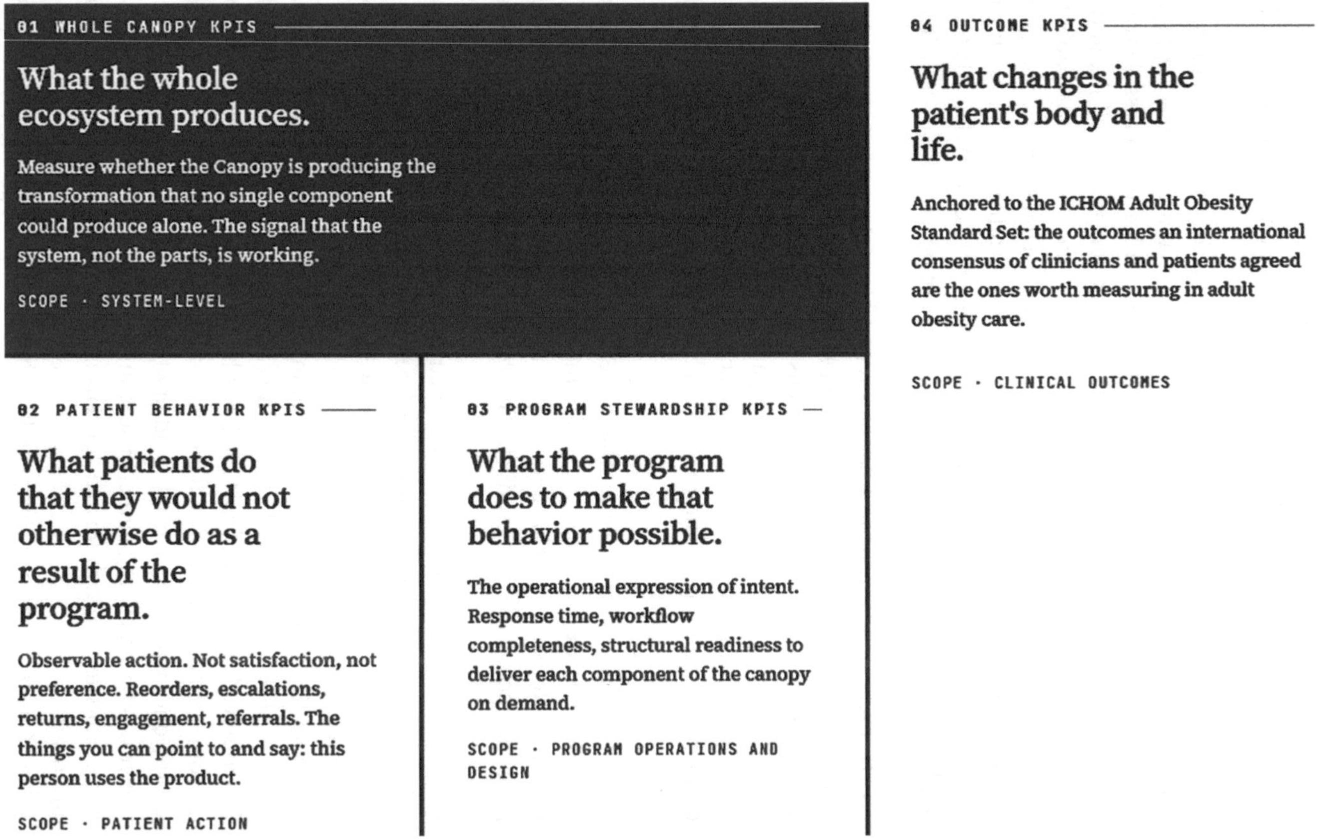

Figure 9.2 The Canopy framework KPI areas.

The architecture is standardized enough that any two programs can be compared on the same metric, and malleable enough to accommodate the regulatory, jurisdictional, and product variation the obesity medicine market will see over the next decade. A cash-pay direct-to-consumer program and an employer-sponsored benefit platform both need to answer the same underlying question: Are patients transforming? The Canopy framework KPIs let them answer it without answering it in identical ways.

Within each component level, KPIs are organized into two tiers. In my practice, a shift occurs around day 30. The patient who comes back for month two is not the same patient who walked in on day one.

The *experience tier* covers the first 30 days. The question at this tier is whether the patient successfully entered the system. Did the order arrive, and did they reorder? Was clinical onboarding completed? Did they encounter the curriculum? Did they meet a coach? Did they enter the community? Did monitoring begin? The experience tier closes with the patient's decision to engage with the second month of the program.

The *engagement tier* covers the period from month two to month 12. Are they using the parts of the system that are supposed to keep them in a state of transformation? Are they self-initiating contact when they need to? Are they sustaining data sharing? Are they learning at the moments that matter?

Each component carries two patient behavior KPIs and two program stewardship KPIs across these two tiers, 14 of each at the C level. Then comes the third tier, where we measure the Canopy itself.

WHY EMPOWERMENT LIVES IN THE WHOLE CANOPY

Empowerment is the last stage of transformation. It is the patient at month 14 who has stopped thinking of the program as a program and started thinking of themselves as someone with a chronic disease they are managing. They self-monitor and advocate for themselves. They know which side-effect responses to try before reaching out. They have integrated their treatment into their lives.

The shift can be seen in where the patient locates themselves in relation to the program. At the experience tier, a patient can say, "I am trying this thing." At the engagement tier, a patient can say, "I am growing inside this thing." At the empowerment tier, a patient can say, "I have found within myself a new identity that exists outside this thing." The program becomes an infrastructure that the patient moves through rather than a project the patient works on.

You cannot attribute that to any one component. You cannot say it was the coaching, the curriculum, or the community; it was all of them together producing a result that no single component could produce alone.

Empowerment tier KPIs measure the system. There are 18 of them. Four are patient behavior KPIs that detect observable signatures of a transformed patient. Four are program stewardship KPIs that detect whether the program was structurally designed to produce transformation in the first place. And ten are outcome KPIs drawn from the ICHOM set as whole Canopy measures.

In total, there are 50 KPIs on the menu (see Figure 9.3). No one program needs to use all of them. But to say your business works at scale over the long term, you need evidence of patients moving from experience to engagement to empowerment. Without it, you have solved for the *wrong* last mile.

TWO EXAMPLE KPIS

You will learn more about each KPI in the following chapters. What I want to share here is the logic behind the KPIs as well as how adaptable they are across different contexts. Consider the following two different KPIs.

First reorder rate (KPI 1) is a patient behavior KPI that measures the patient's willingness to pay the cost of the program for the second time (see Figure 9.4). If the program is mostly medication, did the patient order another month of medication? The second payment event is the closest thing in the data to a vote of confidence. It means that they realized value for the price they paid. The metric is malleable to the product, but the underlying signal is the same: a patient who reorders has decided, with their own money and their own time, that the first round was worth doing again.

Organic referral rate (KPI 36) is a patient behavior KPI that marks the empowerment phase of the transformation (see Figure 9.5). It reflects the patient's endorsement-by-referral of the whole system, not just one component. The organic referral rate is the strongest behavioral signature of empowerment because it indicates that the patient is taking the program into their world and is sharing it with their communities.

The Canopy framework is developed across Chapters 10 through 17, with each chapter introducing the metrics it covers and showing how they are constructed.

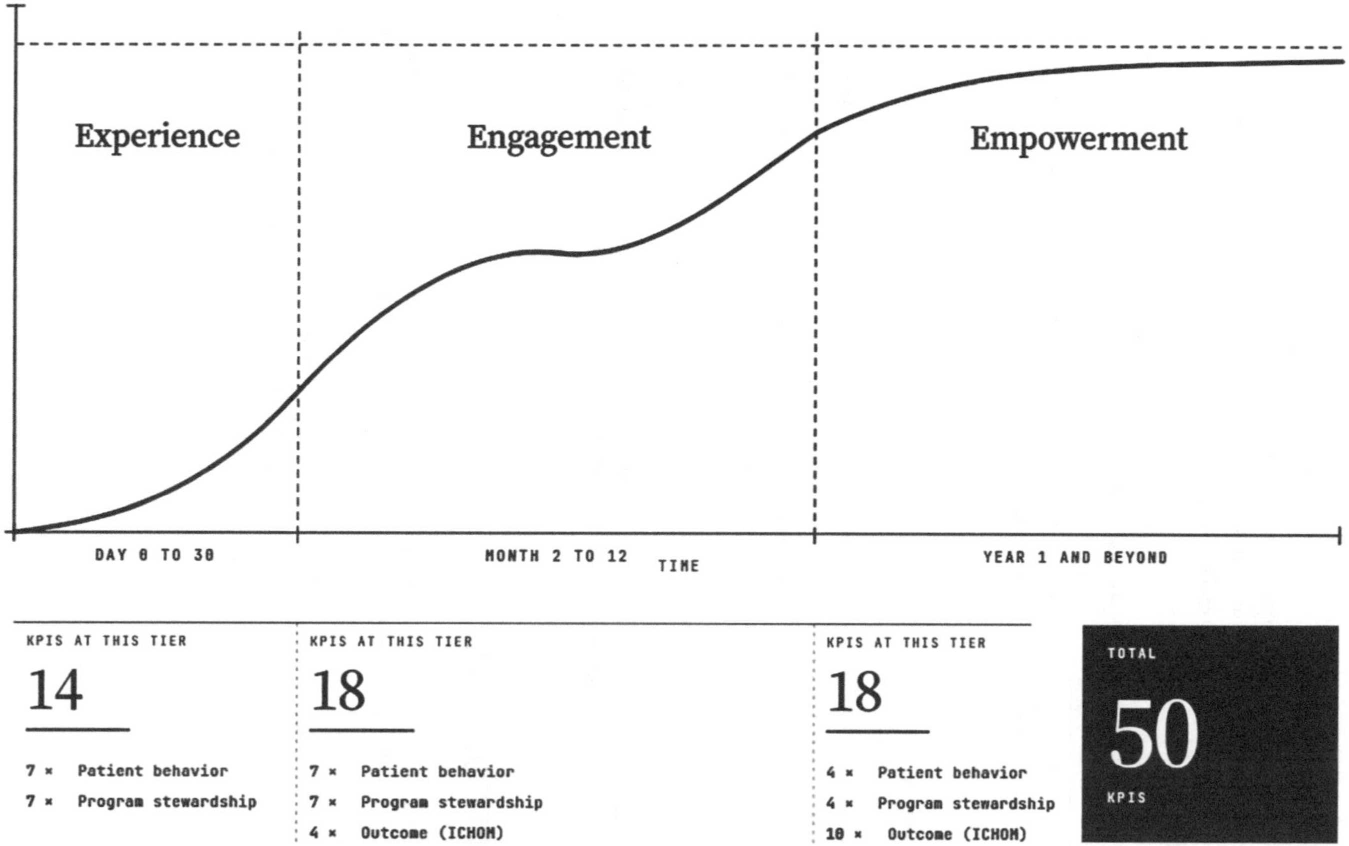

Figure 9.3 The Canopy framework KPI system.

COMPONENT **COST** LENS **PATIENT BEHAVIOR** TIER **EXPERIENCE** **KPI 01 OF 50**

KPI 1, First reorder rate. **The percentage of enrolled patients who place or authorize a second order within 30 to 45 days of the initial order. It is the earliest revealed-preference signal that the patient perceived the price as defensible against the experience of the first month: the first psychological pricing threshold cleared.**

TIMEFRAME **Day 30 to day 45 after first order.**

Figure 9.4 First reorder rate KPI. See Chapter 10 for the full measurement protocol, signal interpretation, and reorder-window rationale.

COMPONENT **SYSTEM** LENS **PATIENT BEHAVIOR** TIER **EMPOWERMENT** **KPI 36 OF 50**

KPI 36, Organic referral rate. **The share of new enrollments in a given month attributable to referrals from existing patients with no incentive, credit, or reward attached. It is the latest revealed-preference signal that the program is working: unprompted referral as a signature of ongoing transformation, and a rising rate indicates that patients have overcome enough shame to share.**

TIMEFRAME **Monthly, with a rolling 12-month trailing rate.**

Figure 9.5 Organic referral rate KPI. See Chapter 17 for the full measurement protocol, signal interpretation, and referral-attribution rationale.

WHAT FOLLOWS

The following chapters are for the builders and system-thinkers among us. You see that most consumer experiences will change as AI moves us away from linear, deterministic work. This means that we get to build better systems—ones that help people do the hard work of personal transformation. But you need a way to communicate your vision and design for the near future and measure your success relative to monocrops. Each chapter in Part III explains how.

ENDNOTES

1. Capgemini Research Institute, *The Last-Mile Delivery Challenge: Giving Retail and Consumer Product Customers a Superior Delivery Experience Without Impacting Profitability* (2019), https://www.capgemini.com/wp-content/uploads/2019/01/Report-Digital-%E2%80%93-Last-Mile-Delivery-Challenge1.pdf; Caroline Hassett, "Last-Mile Delivery Statistics and Industry Insights 2025," SmartRoutes, October 9, 2025, https://smartroutes.io/blogs/last-mile-delivery-statistics-the-complete-data-resource/.
2. Nicholas Economides, "The Economics of the Internet Backbone," *Elsevier B.V.*, Handbook of Telecommunications Economics, vol. 2 (2005): 375, 393–94, https://doi.org/10.1016/S1569-4045(05)02009-9.
3. Mariyam Jameela, "The 7 Rs of Logistics and Supply Chain Management: Key Principles Explained," *WareIQ*, July 14, 2025, https://wareiq.com/resources/blogs/the-7-rs-of-logistics-and-supply-chain/.
4. Steve Banker, "A Critical Fulfillment Metric: The Perfect Order," *Logistics Viewpoints*, November 10, 2014, https://logisticsviewpoints.com/2014/11/10/a-critical-fulfillment-metric-the-perfect-order/.
5. "Hims & Hers Health, Inc. Reports Fourth Quarter and Full Year 2024 Financial Results," Hims & Hers, 2024, https://investors.hims.com/news/news-details/2025/Hims--Hers-Health-Inc.-Reports-Fourth-Quarter-and-Full-Year-2024-Financial-Results/.
6. Jason M. Samuels et al., "Real-World Titration, Persistence & Weight Loss of Semaglutide and Tirzepatide in an Academic Obesity Clinic," *Diabetes, Obesity and Metabolism* 27, no. 11 (2025): 6200–209, https://doi.org/10.1111/dom.70004.
7. Suzanne W. Simard et al., "Net Transfer of Carbon between Ectomycorrhizal Tree Species in the Field," *Nature* 388, no. 6642 (August 7, 1997): 579–82, https://doi.org/10.1038/41557.
8. International Consortium for Health Outcomes Measurement, "Adult Obesity," *ICHOM*, n.d., accessed May 9, 2026, https://www.ichom.org/patient-centered-outcome-measure/adult-obesity/.

CHAPTER 10

COST IN THE CANOPY

Wayne is sitting at the desk in the corner of his home office on a Thursday afternoon. There are two browser tabs open on his laptop. Each one shows a different digital obesity program. Since he stopped taking semaglutide the last time, he has regained all 15 pounds. He is frustrated that he can't get the weight loss to stick, and his blood sugar numbers are back to prediabetes levels. He knows he needs to try again, but has lost confidence in his family doctor to help him through the hard parts.

The first tab shows a program that appeared when he typed *cheap Ozempic* into the Google search bar. It offers the medication for $249 a month, sent to an online pharmacy after a short questionnaire, with no waiting for a doctor's appointment and automatic refills. The second tab shows a program that his colleague Tom recommended after losing 40 pounds last year. At $299 a month, it offers all the same features, plus weekly coach check-ins, a resource library of patient-friendly videos on side effects and meal planning, and 24/7 direct messaging with a pharmacist and a nurse. The second program seems helpful.

Wayne is not sure that the extra $50 is worth it. An additional $600 annual line item is substantial. The semaglutide alone stretches his budget. The extra support may be a luxury, but not a necessity. He clicks back to the $249 tab. He has given himself injections before. He has managed his other medications for years without anyone checking in. He does not think of himself as a person who needs coaching. He hovers over the checkout button. Then he closes the laptop without clicking. He will decide later.

Fifty dollars per month funds transformation infrastructure that will help Wayne succeed for decades. He is medically complex, and the medication-only program is too fragile to support him. But Wayne can't perceive the added value based on a website.

Chapter 9 described the Canopy as an integrated system of seven components and showed why a program built around a single component produces a weak monocrop. This chapter takes the first of the seven components and asks what it means to design it for patient success. Cost is the component that determines the economic envelope within which all other components operate.

PRODUCT-PRICE FIT

The public conversation on obesity medications is dominated by messaging about the lowest possible price. This is important. But there is a missing question too: "What price point, charged to whom, in what mix of cash and coverage, can fund the construction and operation of transformation infrastructure at a quality level that produces clinical outcomes for that segment of patients?" That is a pricing architecture question. It produces a different number, applied differently to different patients, resulting in different downstream behaviors that a company can measure.

In their book *Monetizing Innovation*, Madhavan Ramanujam and Georg Tacke call this product-price fit.[1] *Product-market fit* asks whether the product solves some type of problem. *Product-price fit* asks whether the product, at its current price, provides enough value for the customer to renew willingly and increase spending over time. The first is necessary for a company to exist. The second is what allows compound growth. The obesity programs that survive the next five years are the ones that achieve product-price fit within the program ecosystem, not just product-market fit for the medication.

This is the move from market share to wallet share described in Chapter 3. Hims & Hers counts new starts and reports them quarterly. A wallet-share company counts how much of a patient's ongoing healthcare spend in the obesity category it captures and how much of that spend the patient willingly renews.

THE FOUR COST COMPONENT KPIS

The four component-level key performance indicators (KPIs) for Cost indicate whether the pricing architecture is producing the behaviors we know show up in a transforming patient. Two KPIs measure patient behavior, and two KPIs measure program stewardship.

In my practice, I know a patient has cleared the first threshold when they come back to see me. I do not rely on net promoter scores or satisfaction surveys because patient behavior matters more. I know the threshold is passed with the second order. The second payment event is the closest thing in the data to a real vote of confidence.

The first reorder rate (see KPI 1) produces a binary signal before anything else does: The patient either reordered or did not. A reorder does not indicate *why* the patient came back. The companion program stewardship KPI captures the reason.

Discovery rate (see KPI 2) is the program stewardship companion to the first reorder rate. The first reorder rate indicates whether the patient returned. The discovery rate indicates whether the patient found what was waiting for them. A low discovery rate is a near-term predictor of a future disengagement.

The experience tier KPIs focus on creating a balanced first impression and setting the stage for an ongoing relationship. The engagement tier, which runs from month two through month twelve, indicates whether that early experience has become something worth paying for while giving the program time to support the underlying transformation.

Service gross revenue retention (GRR) separates medication revenue, which is shaped by external pricing pressure and middlemen dynamics, from the service revenue, which is shaped by the transformation infrastructure (see KPI 3). A program with a high service GRR offers value to patients that helps the medication do its job. Each company can set its own thresholds for each KPI, but the framework allows comparison of transformation infrastructure as different as apples and oranges.

Public software-as-a-service (SaaS) companies routinely report gross revenue retention (the share of existing subscription revenue that renews from one period to the next, excluding new sales) in the high eighties to low nineties, with the median clustered around 90%.[2] Programs operating in obesity medicine should be aiming for the same.

Every day or week, patients decide whether to abandon their treatment or continue with it. A program that simply connects a patient to a prescription will not support this decision in real time. A bad week, a cash-flow squeeze, or a moment of doubt may cause them to throw their hands up in exasperation and quit.

If left to their own devices, patients struggle to reconcile the cost of medication with the opportunity cost of side effects, the disappointment at still having to pay attention to their meal structure, and finding time to move their body. Patients believe they were promised a miracle. But medicine does not work that way. A comprehensive, multicomponent program helps patients acquire a balanced view of the costs and benefits of stopping or continuing. The program components engage their values and fears, as well as their need for belonging and care. This helps them make the right decision for themselves and, if the transformation is underway, they usually persist.

Programs should allow their patients to fill prescriptions at any pharmacy they choose, but vertically integrated pharmacies attached to clinical programs usually

KPI 01 OF 50

COMPONENT	LENS	TIER
COST	**PATIENT BEHAVIOR**	**EXPERIENCE**

KPI **FIRST REORDER RATE**

The percentage of enrolled patients who place or authorize a second order within 30 to 45 days of the initial order.

MEASURES	Whether each patient in an enrollment cohort returned for the second month, counted as a percentage of the whole cohort. The day-30-to-day-45 window allows for normal dosing titration without penalizing late-arriving second orders.
SIGNAL	The earliest revealed-preference signal that the patient perceived the price as defensible against the experience of the first month. A patient who reorders has cleared the first psychological pricing threshold: the experience was worth repeating at least once at this price.
TIMEFRAME	Day 30 to day 45 after the first order.

KPI 02 OF 50

COMPONENT	LENS	TIER
COST	**PROGRAM STEWARDSHIP**	**EXPERIENCE**

KPI **DISCOVERY RATE**

The percentage of available program components that the patient has touched at least once by day 30.

MEASURES	Whether the onboarding flow surfaced the full offer to the patient, counted as a cohort-averaged share. The count includes only patient-initiated or patient-responsive events (clicks, attended sessions, opens, replies, submissions), not auto-delivered notifications.
SIGNAL	A patient who has touched every component in the first 30 days knows what they've paid for. This is a critical early retention signal.
TIMEFRAME	Day 0 to day 30 after enrollment.

KPI 03 OF 50

COMPONENT	LENS	TIER
COST	**PATIENT BEHAVIOR**	**ENGAGEMENT**

KPI **SERVICE GRR**

For a patient cohort in a given measurement month, the fraction of the prior month's non-medication service revenue that survived into the current month, excluding expansion revenue. In plain language: of the money the program was collecting last month for the components, how much of it is still coming in this month?

MEASURES	The durability of willingness to pay for the services across months two to twelve, separated from the revenue generated by the medication. Expansion from volume growth and tier upgrades is excluded, so the number is not flattered by growth.
SIGNAL	The revealed-preference willingness-to-pay metric for the service bundle, independent of drug pricing. When willingness to pay for the components stays above its price, patients renew and Service GRR is positive. When willingness to pay drops below price, patients downgrade or cancel and Service GRR declines.
TIMEFRAME	Monthly, across months two through twelve of the patient cohort.

offer better prices to cash-paying patients. Any amount the program charges above the medication cost is used to fund everything else. A monthly payment of $50 per patient, applied across the components, funds the thinnest version of the Canopy: asynchronous messaging, a Curriculum library, and asynchronous Coaching touchpoints. With a monthly payment of $100, even more services would be available.

THE FLYWHEEL OF SUCCESS

Intelligent, early investment in patient success creates a transformation that leads to organic referrals and long-term retention. This lowers the cost of acquisition, so profit grows even as more is invested in transformation infrastructure. Long-term patients have a lower cost to serve, which also improves margins. This is wallet share in action, and here is how it works in the era of medication price compression.

It starts at *discovery*. A patient who finds their way to multiple components within the first 30 days has a willingness to pay that is anchored in several sources of value rather than in a single one. That willingness shows up in the first reorder rate, which remains high, giving the program a runway to reach the longer-horizon metrics. By month three, the depth rate (see KPI 4) begins to climb as the patient builds a routine around two or three components. By month six, the cohort's service GRR has stabilized in the high nineties, because the patients who would have left while on the medication alone have stayed for the transformation they understand is underway. By month 12, the multicomponent cohort renews at rates exceeding those of medication-only cohorts. This creates a second and third year of revenue from patients it would otherwise have had to replace.

The replacement patient requires a fresh acquisition investment each time, whereas keeping the retained patient costs almost nothing additional. A company with a high retention rate is converting its initial acquisition investment into compounding returns because of the transformation. A company with a high discontinuation rate is paying the acquisition cost again every year, which is to say it is running on an acquisition treadmill that speeds up as the price of the molecule comes down and competitors enter the same channel.

The flywheel also produces secondary effects. A transformed patient refers others, and referred patients are 16% more valuable than patients acquired through paid media, plus they stay longer.[3] The cohort that the flywheel produces generates its own acquisition channel, at no marginal cost. Transformed patients are also more likely to expand into adjacent services as their needs evolve: different diagnostics, new treatment areas, coaching for new life phases, and support through stresses that derail adherence. Each expansion adds revenue without adding acquisition cost. This is what you're building toward and what the KPIs measure.

KPI 04 OF 50

COMPONENT	LENS	TIER
COST	**PROGRAM STEWARDSHIP**	**ENGAGEMENT**

KPI **DEPTH RATE**

The average number of distinct available components each active patient meaningfully engages with per month, trended across months two to 12.

MEASURES	The depth of a patient's functional relationship with the bundle, expressed as an average count of distinct components used per active patient per month. The meaningful-engagement threshold is specified per component.
SIGNAL	The wallet-share formation metric. Multi-component engagement is the most replicated retention predictor in subscription economics.
TIMEFRAME	Monthly, across months two to twelve of the patient cohort.

Your attention should be on answering, "Which components produce willingness to pay for more than medication fees, and how much of the available margin should I invest in each of them to produce a service GRR above 90%?" The KPIs provide the metrics to test whether the program is priced correctly and built well. If so, the numbers will rise together. If the program has overbuilt or underbuilt, the metrics will disagree, and the disagreement guides iteration. The pricing stops being a guess; it becomes a hypothesis that you can test in real time.

The companies competing on price in medication-only programs can only enter this flywheel of success if they sell compounded medications on which they can retain higher margins than branded ones. In the United States, they're betting that their legal costs do not eat into their profits in 2026. In countries with generic medication, even with in-house pharmacies, the margins on generics are not high enough to support high customer acquisition costs, so the entire business model collapses. Generics also exert downward price pressure on compounded medications in markets where they coexist.

Now is the time to build real programs and spend on components in ways that improve service GRR and depth rate. Patients who have been through the first wave of digital obesity care aren't satisfied with the status quo, but, critically, they are not just asking for cheaper medication; they are asking to be transformed.

KPI GAMES

Every measurement framework eventually faces the temptation to game it. The four KPIs mentioned previously are designed to resist the most obvious forms of gaming, but they are not gaming-proof.

In 2022, Noom paid $62 million to settle a class action lawsuit alleging the company deliberately made cancellation difficult.[4] The case is instructive because a company under pressure to keep service GRR high can do so legitimately, by improving its program so that fewer patients want to cancel—or they can do so illegitimately, by making cancellation harder. Cancellation, downgrading, and pausing should be set up to protect patients. Patients moving on to different programs should be given a simple care plan summary they can take with them.

A program can boost the discovery rate by spamming patients with emails they do not read and by notification bursts in the first 30 days. Discovery rate counts patient-initiated engagement for a reason. Pushed engagement that does not result in patient action is not the signal the metric is trying to capture. The same applies to depth rate. Programs can define their own thresholds for success inside each KPI.

Service GRR and depth rate are cohort-tagged for a reason. A program under pressure can inflate both by excluding complex patients or by reclassifying a patient who has gone quiet as *paused* rather than *discontinued*. The cohort looks better and better on the evaluation dashboard, while the patients who would have benefited most from the program are no longer in it. The defense is to report cohort composition alongside cohort performance.

The KPIs do not tell you how to build what or for whom. They tell you how to test what you do build against what we know will result in the best clinical and commercial outcomes over the long term. A company that builds honestly and reads the metrics honestly will see them rise. A company that builds flimsy monocrop programs will see acquisition costs climb and retention drop.

COMPLEXITY AND THE CANOPY

Wayne's complexity is exactly what makes his enrollment in a long-term wallet-share program work. The trial evidence shows that sustained treatment benefits him more than almost anyone else. The short-horizon monocrops cannot see this. A patient who will renew for 15 or 20 years, at a price that funds what he needs, generates greater lifetime value than patients who reach their goal weight, stabilize, and discontinue even if they shouldn't. Wayne knows he cannot discontinue without consequence. Obesity is not a phase. It is a lifelong condition that lives in the brain, regardless of how the body looks at any given moment.

U.S. CDC (Centers for Disease Control and Prevention) data show that adult obesity prevalence at the lowest income levels reaches roughly 40%, well above the prevalence in the highest income quintiles.[5] The gradient persists even after researchers control for other variables, showing that obesity reflects structural conditions that the price of the medication alone cannot resolve.

There are 80 million Americans in the bottom two income quintiles, making less than $39,000 a year, who cannot pay for obesity medications. The patients who need the most intensive infrastructure are disproportionately those with the fewest economic resources. Pricing has to handle this asymmetry without hiding it or abandoning the patients the monocroppers would screen out. This is where Chapter 11's focus on coverage helps us move beyond prior authorization and into more creative solutions.

Wayne clicks back to the tab with the $299 program. If Wayne's first 30 days in the $299 program produce the components that meet him where he is, he will be able to make an informed decision at that time. If not, he can cancel at month two, confirming his suspicion that the extra cost was a luxury. The program's job in the first 30 days is not to sell Wayne on the value. It is to make the value visible before he must decide whether to pay for it again. Wayne signs up for the pricier program, and the 30-day clock begins.

ENDNOTES

1. Madhavan Ramanujam and Georg Tacke, *Monetizing Innovation: How Smart Companies Design the Product Around the Price* (Hoboken: Wiley, 2016).
2. "2024 SaaS Performance Metrics," Benchmarkit, 2024, https://www.benchmarkit.ai/2024benchmarks.
3. Christophe Van Den Bulte et al., "How Customer Referral Programs Turn Social Capital into Economic Capital," *Journal of Marketing Research* 55, no. 1 (2018): 132–46, https://doi.org/10.1509/jmr.14.0653.
4. Nichols v. Noom, Inc., 1:20-cv-03677-KHP (United States District Court, Southern District of New York, July 12, 2022).
5. "Adult Obesity Facts," Centers for Disease Control and Prevention, May 14, 2024, https://www.cdc.gov/obesity/adult-obesity-facts/index.html; Cynthia L. Ogden et al., "Prevalence of Obesity Among Adults, by Household Income and Education—United States, 2011–2014," *MMWR. Morbidity and Mortality Weekly Report* 66, no. 50 (2017), https://doi.org/10.15585/mmwr.mm6650a1.

CHAPTER 11

COVERAGE IN THE CANOPY

Sarah bounced into her Tuesday morning appointment with me, eight months after I last saw her. The weight she lost in the spring is back. She is thrilled anyway.

"I have a new job," she says, "VP at a different company. The benefits packet hit my inbox yesterday." She turns her phone toward me and scrolls to the formulary. "They cover obesity medications. Not all of them, but semaglutide is on the list. I need your help with the prior authorization form."

I closed her chart. "Tell me what happened after I saw you last."

The compounded semaglutide story I already knew. Her employer had dropped coverage for Wegovy in 2024. We unsuccessfully appealed. She switched to a digital platform to try compounded semaglutide, and then we lost touch. I had not heard the rest of the story. At week nine, she was increased to 1 mg and could not stand the sight of food. By week 10, she was housebound and vomiting. By week 11, she stopped treatment completely—and the weight came back.

I tell her we will fix the coverage and rebuild from there. I also tell her that treating obesity is not just prescribing GLP-1 medications. She mentions that her sleep has not been consistent for months, and her cycle is unpredictable. She is 45 years old. Obesity treatment lives within a broader conversation about chronic disease management, and a good obesity practice is built to hold it all. "Bring all of it back to me," I tell her. "We Care plan for the whole thing."

HOW COVERAGE WORKS

There are four major health insurance coverage categories in the United States. Employer-sponsored insurance covers most working-age Americans (see Figure 11.1). Self-insured employers—the majority of large employers—design their own benefits and bear actual healthcare costs. Employers buy coverage from an insurer that bears the risk. In 2024, 34% of large employers covered GLP-1 medications for weight management.[1] That number has been moving, sometimes upward as employers compete for talent, sometimes downward when utilization exceeds what

01

Employer-sponsored insurance

Coverage tied to a job. Self-insured employers design their own benefits and bear the actual cost of care; fully insured employers buy a plan from a carrier that bears the risk.

GLP-1 TODAY 34% of large employers covered GLP-1s for weight management in 2024; the share moves with the labor market and the budget.

02

Individual marketplace

Plans Americans buy on their own — through healthcare.gov or directly from an insurer — without an employer in the middle. Benefit design varies by carrier and state.

ACCESS ROUTE Open enrollment plus qualifying life events; subsidies for households under defined income thresholds.

03

Public coverage

Medicare for Americans 65 and over, Medicaid for low-income Americans, plus VA and Tricare for veterans and military families. Each program writes its own rules for obesity medications.

STATUTE Medicare's 2003 law bars coverage of drugs "for weight loss"; access today runs through cardiovascular and sleep-apnea indications and the 2026 BALANCE demonstration.

04

Direct cash-pay

The patient pays out of pocket, increasingly through a manufacturer storefront that sells branded medication outside the insurance system at below the list price.

EXAMPLES *LillyDirect* and *NovoCare* — branded channels operated by Eli Lilly and Novo Nordisk.

Figure 11.1 Four coverage categories in the United States.

budgets were built to absorb. North Carolina's State Health Plan for its employees dropped GLP-1 coverage for obesity in April 2024 after projecting a $1 billion exposure over six years.[2]

The second coverage category is the individual marketplace, where Americans buy plans through *healthcare.gov* or directly from an insurer. The third category is public coverage: Medicare for Americans 65 and over, Medicaid for low-income Americans, as well as VA and Tricare for veterans and military families. Medicare's 2003 statute prohibits coverage of medications "for weight loss," which is why a Medicare beneficiary with obesity could receive Wegovy only when the diagnosis was cardiovascular disease or obstructive sleep apnea, both of which the FDA approved in the past two years.[3]

In November 2025, the federal government negotiated a price agreement with Eli Lilly and Novo Nordisk to boost sales volumes and improve access for public beneficiaries. The Centers for Medicare & Medicaid Services (CMS) followed in December 2025 with two demonstrations. The Medicare GLP-1 Bridge is a short-term payment mechanism that lets eligible beneficiaries access these medications for $50 per month. The BALANCE Model is a five-year voluntary pilot designed to extend that same pricing across Medicare Part D and state Medicaid through 2031. The Medicare side of BALANCE stalled in April 2026 when too few Part D plans applied, and CMS extended the Bridge through December 2027 in its place. The Medicaid side of BALANCE is moving forward.[4] Medicaid coverage differs state to state. Sixteen states reported some coverage for obesity in late 2024.[5]

The fourth place is direct cash pay, which is increasingly supported by manufacturers. Examples include LillyDirect and NovoCare, both of which sell branded medications outside the insurance system at much-lower-than-list prices.[6]

Within any of these categories, coverage for a specific medication is governed by a formulary, the insurer's list of covered drugs. Formularies are tiered by cost-sharing. Preferred tier means a lower copay; nonpreferred means a higher copay; nonformulary means the insured patient has to pay cash. Most obesity medications require a prior authorization form. Sarah's form asks me to attest to her need for semaglutide, but, in reality, the form has nothing to do with medical necessity. The forms are simply time-consuming friction that reduces the number of prescriptions the insurers are asked to pay for.

Step therapy sometimes requires the patient to fail on a cheaper drug before the insurer will cover a newer one. When a prior authorization is denied, the patient or clinician can appeal. Peer-to-peer reviews, where a clinician on the platform speaks directly with a clinician at the insurer, sometimes succeed where written appeals do not.

Layered on top of all of this are programs that close the gap between what treatment costs and what the patient can afford. Manufacturer copay cards reduce out-of-pocket costs for commercially insured patients. Patient assistance programs sometimes cover the medication costs in full for patients experiencing financial hardship. Sliding-scale fees—which Federally Qualified Health Centers are required by law to use—adjust the price of clinical services based on income.[7]

COVERAGE IS ACCESS

The Canopy reframes coverage as access to infrastructure. This chapter introduces four KPIs (key performance indicators) to measure how the infrastructure works and incentivizes creativity and coordination. The KPIs work for patients with conventional plans, for patients with no plan, and for cohorts where every patient is price-sensitive.

Each new patient needs their own funding plan. The coverage acceptance rate (see KPI 5) captures their acceptance of the plan. A patient who enters the coverage-determination workflow, sees a documented funding plan that makes sense for them, and proceeds into the program has resolved many of the *what-if?* worries that patients have on day one. This is a standard-setting experience for patients and demonstrates that they are working with experts who care about their budget as much as they do.

The companion measure is the time the program takes to get a patient from workflow entry to a documented funding plan they can actually accept (see KPI 6). A funding plan for someone paying cash could take just a few seconds to build. It is the same for a patient who wants to pay cash and seek reimbursement later. It could take days to weeks to build a funding plan for a patient who needs to use their insurance.

Ro CEO Zachariah Reitano said the cost burden and the insurance navigation burden were the two reasons patients did not even take the first step.[8] Ro's response was to build an insurance coverage checker that patients could use before committing to a clinical relationship. Ro understands that coverage navigation can be a moat rather than just friction to be avoided.

The engagement tier is more complicated. Sarah's employer dropping coverage in week six of treatment is common. So are job changes, formulary switches, prior-authorization lapses, copay tier increases, or expiring manufacturer assistance programs. Affordability events arrive in every cohort. The most price-sensitive patients are vulnerable to dropping out from these events. But if the program demonstrates competent coverage navigation in the first month, then the patient who needs help after a budget shock will reach out.

How do you tell which patients are price-sensitive? Program designers can embed direct measures into their user journey, but these can also be inferred from coverage type, occupation, preferences, behavior, and free-text inputs collected from

KPI 05 OF 50

COMPONENT	LENS	TIER
COVERAGE	**PATIENT BEHAVIOR**	**EXPERIENCE**

KPI **COVERAGE ACCEPTANCE RATE**

The percentage of patients who accept the funding plan presented to them and proceed into the program.

MEASURES

Patients who accepted a documented funding plan, whether insurance-verified or cash-pay with applicable assistance layered on, and proceeded to at least one forward step (such as first service payment authorized), divided by all patients who entered the coverage-determination workflow.

SIGNAL

A high rate indicates that the coverage component matches the population the program enrolls. A low rate means the program is signing up patients it cannot actually treat.

TIMEFRAME

Day 0 to Day 30 from workflow entry, reported by monthly enrollment cohort.

KPI 06 OF 50

COMPONENT	LENS	TIER
COVERAGE	**PROGRAM STEWARDSHIP**	**EXPERIENCE**

KPI **TIME-TO-ACCEPTANCE**

The median number of hours from a patient's entry into the coverage-determination workflow to acceptance of a documented funding plan.

MEASURES

Hours from workflow-entry timestamp to funding-plan acceptance timestamp, calculated as a median across each monthly cohort.

SIGNAL

A short and stable median means the classification and routing machinery works for most patients. A long or rising median, or a wide gap between median and the 90th percentile, means there is a lot of coverage-related friction.

TIMEFRAME

Reported monthly; report median and 90th percentile, compared across primary funding types.

other workflows. Patients will write things like, "I was getting my Ozempic from this company, but then they raised their fees, so I came here to check out your fees." That is a price-sensitive patient.

Understanding patients' financial situation is table stakes for clinicians, as it should be for any program wanting to scale across markets. Just as I keep a record of my patients' medical histories, I also know their coverage and socioeconomic status. It is part of the treatment plan, so it must be part of the Canopy. I am intimately familiar with the rebates available, how to make medications last longer, and how to optimize everything else to keep GLP-1 doses as low as possible. I write battle-ready prior authorization forms. I am in the affordability thicket with my patients, especially the ones paying cash.

Many companies want to opt out of coverage navigation because it seems complex and labor-intensive. Given the choice between spending a few hours of a customer service representative's time on coverage navigation or spending many hundreds of dollars on paid ads to re-acquire that customer, I choose the labor for someone this far down the funnel. The labor makes an impression, establishes a relationship, and sets up wallet share. Labor can be well supported by effective automation, making their job much smoother.

Price sensitivity is not the same as being poor. Some low-income patients may have very stable medication coverage and are less sensitive to medication pricing than to program pricing. Some are price-sensitive because they live close to their margin, and a $50 swing is the difference between retention and dropout. Some are price-sensitive because their coverage is unstable, and any affordability event could change their out-of-pocket math. Some are price-sensitive at the moment because of divorce, a job change, or a hospitalization that drained their savings. Some are just very frugal by nature, or perhaps nurture. The retention parity ratio (see KPI 7) is intentionally inclusive.

The fourth metric measures whether the program can detect price-pressure signals and act on them. A patient about to lose coverage or skip a payment may offer a signal before dropping out. The signal might be a declined transaction, a downgrade attempt, a cancellation inquiry, a pause request, or an expiring assistance program. Patients struggle to directly ask for help with affordability (see KPI 8—affordability response rate). Programs may have an affordability support chat feature to make it easier for patients to request help.

The metrics do not demand charity. But they do reward up-front investments in a patient's lifetime value. Patients invest their trust in programs early because they have to. That trust is step one toward wallet-share territory. Dumping the therapeutic relationship after an affordability event is both unethical and commercially irrational.

KPI 07 OF 50

COMPONENT	LENS	TIER
COVERAGE	**PATIENT BEHAVIOR**	**ENGAGEMENT**

KPI **RETENTION PARITY RATIO**

The ratio of 12-month active retention in the price-sensitive cohort to 12-month active retention in the whole cohort.

MEASURES	Price-sensitive 12-month retention divided by whole cohort 12-month retention, expressed as a ratio. The price-sensitive cohort is defined inclusively: patients who enrolled in a manufacturer assistance program at signup, selected the lowest-priced program tier, had a declined transaction on file, downgraded within 90 days, requested a payment plan, or skipped a service payment month. Programs can instill other stable measures of price-sensitivity into their workflow.
SIGNAL	A ratio at or near 1.0 means the dynamic-affordability machinery is working, and price-sensitive patients are staying at the same rate as everyone else.
TIMEFRAME	12-month retention measured cohort-over-cohort.

KPI 08 OF 50

COMPONENT	LENS	TIER
COVERAGE	**PROGRAM STEWARDSHIP**	**ENGAGEMENT**

KPI **AFFORDABILITY RESPONSE RATE**

The percentage of patients showing a price-pressure signal who receive a meaningful affordability intervention within seven days.

MEASURES	Patients who received a meaningful affordability intervention (downwards tier adjustment of at least 20 percent, pause of at least 30 days, new assistance program enrollment, payment plan, or coverage bridge supply) within seven days of a flagged signal, divided by all price-pressure signals detected in the period.
SIGNAL	A high rate means the detection-and-response loop has formed. A low rate means response is late or non-existent.
TIMEFRAME	Reported monthly, measured against a seven-day response window from signal detection.

CREATIVE COVERAGE

Wayne has no insurance. He is not poor enough for Medicaid, he does not meet the retirement requirements for Medicare, and he has no employer-sponsored plan. His semaglutide is the most expensive health line item on his monthly budget.

For Wayne, *coverage* is whatever is available. Cash-pay through direct-to-consumer pricing keeps the medication itself within reach at compressed prices. Manufacturer assistance programs can help, but are not always stable. The older patient assistance programs were originally designed for the uninsured, but now eligibility is income-tested. Wayne's small business income lands him in an awkward bracket: too high for hardship, yet too low to absorb $299 a month for the rest of his life.

Three creative coverage mechanisms expand the addressable market to include patients like Wayne. Income-based pricing adjusts the program's service fee based on the patient's ability to pay. Federally Qualified Health Centers (FQHCs) have used sliding fee scales for decades because they are required to do so under Health Resources and Services Administration policy.[9] A platform that offers obesity treatment at $299 a month for full pay and $199 for documented financial need captures both populations under the same clinical protocol, with infrastructure costs spread across more patients. The legal framework for income-based cost-sharing is well established. Any program that is serious about widening its addressable market should use it.[10]

Value-based arrangements tie payment directly to clinical outcomes. Programs could accept a reduced up-front payment in exchange for an additional payment when defined clinical milestones are achieved, such as 5% weight loss maintained at 12 months, mirroring the value-based structures Novo Nordisk and Eli Lilly have established with payers.[11] The mechanism works when there is an alternative payer who wants to limit its downside. When the payer is the patient, there is a moral hazard to defend against. A patient could under-report their success to avoid the additional payment. Creative and collaborative coverage options include:

1. FQHCs already use sliding fee scales and are required to serve patients regardless of their ability to pay. An FQHC could partner with a digital obesity platform under a value-based arrangement in which the platform absorbs the up-front infrastructure cost and the FQHC shares documented savings from reduced emergency visits and hospitalizations. Wayne's prediabetes, hypertension, and cardiovascular risk make him exactly the patient whose downstream costs are highest if untreated.
2. State Medicaid programs are increasingly experimenting with Section 1115 waivers that cover obesity treatment. A value-based arrangement with a state Medicaid organization could tie the second payment to documented

clinical milestones (A1c below 6.0, blood pressure at target, and/or sustained weight loss) rather than to weight loss alone. Several states have approved GLP-1 coverage under these waivers, and the Medicaid track of the BALANCE Model signals that CMS is engaging directly with state programs on coordinated GLP-1 coverage architectures.[12]

3. Employer-adjacent arrangements for the self-employed are worth exploring. Wayne runs a small business with two employees. Small business health purchasing cooperatives and association health plans could pool risk across thousands of small employers to negotiate group rates for obesity treatment programs.[13] The platform offers a lower per-member price in exchange for guaranteed volume.
4. Nonprofit hospitals are required under federal law to conduct a triennial community health needs assessment and adopt an implementation strategy to address identified priorities, and large charitable organizations like the American Heart Association direct substantial grant funding toward community health improvement.[14] A value-based partnership where the foundation funds the first 90 days of treatment and the platform continues at reduced cost if the patient hits clinical milestones creates a shared-risk model that serves uninsured patients without requiring either party to absorb all the cost.

Coverage bridges are temporary subsidies that hold the patient in treatment while a primary coverage path comes back online. When an employer drops coverage, when a job changes, or when a prior authorization lapses during an appeal, a coverage bridge keeps the medication flowing. The platform absorbs short-term cost in exchange for preserving a relationship that would otherwise end, and the cost of the bridge is typically well below the cost of reacquiring the patient. The best bridges are automatic, triggered by detected changes in coverage status, with a defined duration and a clear handoff to permanent resolution. They are captured in the affordability response rate.

For Wayne, the creative path looks like this. His funding plan confirms the lowest direct-to-consumer price available.[15] The coverage team enrolls him in the manufacturer assistance program for the months his quarterly income drops. It sets a 60-day formulary watch on the manufacturer announcements that change cash pricing in either direction. It bundles his obesity care with the rest of his chronic disease management and derives revenue from his whole picture. Nothing revolutionary here, but it requires a coverage team that treats his cash-pay status as a strategic path to long-term retention.

The harder case is the cohort where every patient is price-sensitive at once. A program serving a Medicaid expansion population, a community health center contracting for obesity care, or a rural employer plan with a small workforce will see the retention parity ratio collapse, not because the price-sensitive cohort is being abandoned, but because the entire cohort is price-sensitive. The single full-price tier does not work as the main offer. A no-frills version of the Canopy with a low monthly fee has to be the main offer. To get price-product fit, the program must be designed around what public coverage already pays for. Revenue comes from volume that must be retained. Success here is possible but requires operational mastery and creativity.

For Medicare beneficiaries specifically, there are pathways forward for programs that design for this population. Medicare does not yet pay for obesity medication outside the GLP-1 Bridge, which runs through December 2027, but it does pay for primary care visits, lab work, cardiology and endocrinology referrals, and the chronic disease management codes that enable obesity care. A program serving cash-pay seniors can route the medication through manufacturer programs or the Bridge at $50 per month for eligible patients, while routing all other clinical work through Medicare-covered visits and labs. Broader coverage for evidence-based obesity treatment is essential. Programs that build tenable practice models will be viable partners for future Medicare expansion.

THE LONG GAME FOR COVERAGE

The longer-term economic case for better system-wide coverage infrastructure is growing rapidly. Thorpe and Joski found that commercially insured patients who achieved 5% weight loss showed average annual reductions in healthcare spending of approximately $670 per patient, and patients who achieved 25% weight loss showed reductions of approximately $2,849 per patient annually.[16] The savings scale with the weight loss, which means every incremental percentage point a program delivers translates directly into reduced downstream spending. Those savings accrue to whoever pays for downstream care: patients with high deductibles, self-insured employers, and, over time, to the government. Medicare and Medicaid are the longest-tenure payers in this market. They cover populations whose obesity prevalence is rising fastest; the Congressional Budget Office estimates that 34% of all Part D enrollees currently have obesity, with the prevalence climbing toward 47% by 2030.[17]

At the negotiated $245 monthly Medicare price, obesity medications cost between $53,400 and $61,400 per quality-adjusted life year, well below the $100,000 to $150,000 range the United States typically pays for chronic disease prevention.[18] BALANCE was supposed to be the federal test of whether broader GLP-1 coverage could pay for itself. The Medicare side stalled in April 2026 when insurers, unable to predict how many beneficiaries would continue taking the medications, declined to assume the risk. The system cannot underwrite coverage at scale until it has confidence in the delivery infrastructure that determines who stays on treatment. The GLP-1 Bridge now carries the data-collection burden through 2027. If the Bridge produces persistence and outcomes strong enough to shift insurer expectations, broader Medicare coverage becomes negotiable. If it does not, the 2003 exclusion holds. Either way, the government has the most to gain from working coverage and the longest time horizon over which to capture it.

FROM COVERAGE TO CARE

Sarah's new employer's formulary is quickly analyzed by the Coverage agent I built and trained to support my team's human reimbursement specialist. It flags semaglutide as preferred-tier with a prior authorization requirement and produces a funding plan: $50 monthly copay, with a manufacturer copay card layered on for the first six months. The reimbursement specialist reviews for accuracy and finalizes it. The provisional funding plan reaches Sarah's inbox before our next visit. She accepted her funding plan in under 24 hours.

The prior authorization itself is completed by the agent, reviewed by the specialist, and sent to me for final human-in-the-loop review and signature. Sarah's prior authorization is approved on a Thursday. Her medication ships the same day from her preferred pharmacy and arrives on Friday. Sarah's first injection is Monday morning, six days after she walked back into my office.

ENDNOTES

1. *Employee Benefits Survey: 2024 Survey Report*, Survey Report (International Foundation of Employee Benefit Plans, 2024), https://www.ifebp.org/detail-pages/resource/survey/employee-benefits-survey--2024-survey-report.
2. North Carolina State Health Plan for Teachers and State Employees, "Board of Trustees Meeting Minutes," April 25, 2024.
3. Medicare Prescription Drug, Improvement, and Modernization Act of 2003, Pub. L. Nos. 108–173, 42 U.S.C. (2003); "FDA Approves First Treatment to Reduce Risk of Serious Heart Problems Specifically in Adults with Obesity or Overweight," U.S. Food and Drug Administration, FDA, September 8, 2024, https://www.fda.gov/news-events/press-announcements/fda-approves-first-treatment-reduce-risk-serious-heart-problems-specifically-adults-obesity-or; "FDA Approves First Medication for Obstructive Sleep Apnea," FDA News Release, FDA, December 27, 2024, https://www.fda.gov/news-events/press-announcements/fda-approves-first-medication-obstructive-sleep-apnea.
4. The White House, "Fact Sheet: President Donald J. Trump Announces Major Developments in Bringing Most-Favored-Nation Pricing to American Patients," The White House, November 6, 2025, https://www.whitehouse.gov/fact-sheets/2025/11/fact-sheet-president-donald-j-trump-announces-major-developments-in-bringing-most-favored-nation-pricing-to-american-patients/; "CMS Launches Voluntary Model to Expand Access to Life-Changing Medicines, Promote Healthier Living," CMS.Gov, December 23, 2025, https://www.cms.gov/newsroom/press-releases/cms-launches-voluntary-model-expand-access-life-changing-medicines-promote-healthier-living; "BALANCE (Better Approaches to Lifestyle and Nutrition for Comprehensive hEalth) Model," CMS.Gov, April 2026, https://www.cms.gov/priorities/innovation/innovation-models/balance; "Medicare GLP-1 Bridge," CMS.Gov, May 12, 2026, https://www.cms.gov/medicare/coverage/prescription-drug-coverage/medicare-glp-1-bridge; American Hospital Association, "CMS Delays Part D Portion of BALANCE Model on Expansion of GLP-1 Access," American Hospital Association, April 22, 2026, https://www.aha.org/news/headline/2026-04-22-cms-delays-part-d-portion-balance-model-expansion-glp-1-access.
5. "Medicaid Coverage of and Spending on GLP-1s," Kaiser Family Foundation, January 16, 2026, https://www.kff.org/medicaid/medicaid-coverage-of-and-spending-on-glp-1s/.
6. Novo Nordisk, "FDA Approves Novo Nordisk's Wegovy® Pill, the First and Only Oral GLP-1 for Weight Loss in Adults," PR Newswire, December 22, 2025, https://www.prnewswire.com/news-releases/fda-approves-novo-nordisks-wegovy-pill-the-first-and-only-oral-glp-1-for-weight-loss-in-adults-302648344.html; Eli Lilly and Company, "FDA Approves Lilly's Foundayo™ (Orforglipron), the Only GLP-1 Pill for Weight Loss That Can Be Taken Any Time of Day without Food or Water Restrictions," Lilly, April 1, 2026, https://investor.lilly.com/news-releases/news-release-details/fda-approves-lillys-foundayotm-orforglipron-only-glp-1-pill.

7. Health Resources and Services Administration, Bureau of Primary Health Care, "Sliding Fee Discount and Related Billing and Collections Program Requirements," September 22, 2014.
8. Ashley Capoot and Annika Kim Contantino, "Digital Health Company Ro Launches GLP-1 Insurance-Coverage Checker to Help Patients Navigate Costs," CNBC, August 13, 2024, https://www.cnbc.com/2024/08/13/ro-launches-glp-1-insurance-coverage-checker.html.
9. Health Resources and Services Administration, Bureau of Primary Health Care, "Sliding Fee Discount and Related Billing and Collections Program Requirements."
10. Income-based and tiered cost-sharing in group health plans are governed by HIPAA nondiscrimination provisions at ERISA § 702, 29 U.S.C. § 1182, and Public Health Service Act § 2705, 42 U.S.C. § 300gg-4; the self-insured medical reimbursement plan rules at Internal Revenue Code § 105(h), 26 U.S.C. § 105(h); and Affordable Care Act § 2716, codified at 26 U.S.C. § 9815.
11. John Tozzi, "Cigna Strikes Deals with Lilly, Novo for Obesity Coverage," Bloomberg Law, March 7, 2024, https://news.bloomberglaw.com/insurance/cigna-strikes-deals-with-lilly-novo-for-more-obesity-coverage; Bertha Coombs, "Cigna Announces New Deal for Copay Caps on Eli Lilly and Novo Nordisk Weight Loss Drugs," CNBC, May 21, 2025, https://www.cnbc.com/2025/05/21/cigna-eli-lilly-novo-nordisk-weight-loss-drugs.html.
12. "Medicaid Coverage of and Spending on GLP-1s"; CMS.Gov, "BALANCE (Better Approaches to Lifestyle and Nutrition for Comprehensive hEalth) Model."
13. Definition of 'Employer'—Association Health Plans, 89 Federal Register (2024), https://www.federalregister.gov/documents/2024/04/30/2024-08985/definition-of-employer-association-health-plans.
14. Internal Revenue Code § 501(r)(3), 26 U.S.C. § 501(r)(3), and Treas. Reg. § 1.501(r)-3; Internal Revenue Service, "Community Health Needs Assessment for Charitable Hospital Organizations: Section 501(r)(3)," accessed May 2026, https://www.irs.gov/charities-non-profits/community-health-needs-assessment-for-charitable-hospital-organizations-section-501r3.
15. "Online Pharmacy Service Options for Select Lilly Medicines," Lilly Direct®, accessed May 19, 2026, https://www.lilly.com/lillydirect/; "Support Starts Here for Patients Taking Novo Nordisk Medicines," NovoCare®, accessed May 19, 2026, https://www.novocare.com/.
16. Kenneth E. Thorpe and Peter J. Joski, "Estimated Reduction in Health Care Spending Associated with Weight Loss in Adults," *JAMA Network Open* 7, no. 12 (2024): e2449200, https://doi.org/10.1001/jamanetworkopen.2024.49200.
17. *How Would Authorizing Medicare to Cover Anti-Obesity Medications Affect the Federal Budget?* (Congressional Budget Office, 2024), https://www.cbo.gov/publication/60816.
18. Grace A. Lin et al., *Semaglutide and Tirzepatide for Obesity: Effectiveness and Value* (Institute for Clinical and Economic Review, 2025); CMS.Gov, "BALANCE (Better Approaches to Lifestyle and Nutrition for Comprehensive hEalth) Model."

CHAPTER 12

CARE IN THE CANOPY

Wayne sends three documents through his patient portal: (1) a cardiology consultation note from two weeks ago, (2) a pharmacy record of his current medications, and (3) a list of questions from his wife, Linda. He is due for his check-in with the clinical team at the online program he started (mentioned at the end of Chapter 10).

He also has a question of his own. He has been on semaglutide 1 mg weekly for four months. He lost 15 pounds again and then 20 more. He eats three square meals a day without difficulty and doesn't snack much. But his weight has been the same for three weeks, and Linda says 1.7 mg is the next step. He wants to know if he should increase his dose.

Linda recently began semaglutide herself. She became his weekly injection partner, the person who put the medication reminder on the kitchen calendar and kept him on schedule. He is more confident in his treatment plan since they started working on it together.

A clinician who does not prescribe semaglutide regularly would look at Wayne's chart and think:

- He has lost weight on semaglutide
- He has more to lose
- He tolerates the medication
- The monograph says raising the dose to 1.7 mg is the next step

Increase the dose. That is not wrong. But it is incomplete.

Care is the clinical component of the Canopy. Chapters 10 and 11 addressed what the patient pays and whether insurance covers it. This chapter is about what happens next.

Obesity medicine must deliver specialist-level care at the primary care scale. This is a novel and difficult mission. There are over 11,500 board-certified obesity medicine physicians in the United States.[1] There are 126 million adults who meet the clinical criteria for treatment. That ratio cannot be fixed by simply training more specialists. It demands clinical teams with multiple roles, both clinical and non-clinical, to deliver expert-level care under protocol, nested within the Canopy's other components. It requires that the teams be augmented by intelligent protocols and automation, with specialist physicians directing their attention to the patients whose complexity demands it.

The Canopy doesn't exist in most programs. In the digital world, we have mostly monocrop telehealth practices, diet-culture relics, and uncredentialed peptide dealers. We can do far better.

THE MONOCROPPERS

Care and *Curriculum* arise from a rare property in consumer technology: a product that changes how it works as the customer changes. A Peloton bike functions identically whether you have lost zero pounds or 40. A GLP-1 medication does not. As patients lose weight, their metabolism and appetite shift. Doses that worked in month two may be insufficient in month six because the appetite is stronger. Side effects that were tolerable at 0.5 mg may become unmanageable at 1 mg. Someone has to titrate. Someone has to teach the patient what to expect in month four when appetite suppression wanes, so that a normal treatment milestone is not interpreted as the medication failing them. These two components come from real-life clinical practice.

The most common encounter in obesity medicine today happens online. The patient fills out an intake form on a consumer website. They have a brief asynchronous exchange with a clinician or sometimes a brief video visit. They receive a prescription, some emails with medication information, and some basic customer support. When they message for help with side effects, replies are templated and standard: eat smaller meals, drink water, avoid fatty foods, and good luck. If you have a problem, go to the hospital.

These are the monocroppers. Different platforms market themselves with different branding and copy, but the playbook is the same. The business model is built for volume and market share, rather than transformation and wallet share. There is no real Care plan, no specialist coordination, rarely an integrated lab review, no dynamic titration or switching logic that adjusts to the patient's body composition or comorbidities, and no protocol for what to do when appetite suppression has gone too far or not far enough. The medication is the product. The clinician is a regulatory hurdle to be managed, not an expert ally. Everything that should surround the prescription and make it work is absent.

These platforms are not the enemy. In fact, my experiences building clinical protocols for several of these led to this book. The monocroppers have the digital infrastructure, consumer relationships, regulatory experience, and pharmacy distribution that are essential ingredients for long-term success. They do not have a Canopy, but they certainly could build one if they wanted to. The economic argument for doing so is the subject of this book.

Specialists, working inside structured programs that wrap Care around the prescription, hold patients on therapy at meaningfully higher rates than the monocrop model does.[2] Yet specialists write fewer than 10% of obesity medicine prescriptions.[3] The other 90% move through the monocrop pipeline, where the prescription is expected to do work it cannot do.

Prescriptions need Care plans to really benefit patients. Care plans are not made from scratch for every patient. They follow protocols that account for the full range of events a patient's life can throw at treatment: surgery, medication switches, off-label augmentation, dose adjustments as body composition changes, and side-effect management that escalates through defined steps. The protocols also account for the patients whose biology sits outside the typical curve. A patient who had a Roux-en-Y gastric bypass eight years ago and regained 40 pounds responds to GLP-1 therapy differently than a patient on the same dose who has never had surgery, with different risks, appetite physiology, and needs. A patient whose medication response is atypical, or whose hunger never settles even on the maximum dose, may be carrying a rare genetic obesity syndrome. The protocol must ask those questions in a stepwise manner before declaring that the patient simply does not respond to treatment.

Those involved in cancer care figured this out decades ago. Chemotherapy protocols are rigorous and protocolized, including not just the core treatment but also every anticipated complication. Obesity medicine can do the same. Protocol-governed care improves safety, makes costs predictable, and lets the clinical team plan ahead rather than react. The Care plan is a living document. It changes as the patient changes. It is not a prison. It is a scaffold that holds the treatment together while the patient changes over time.

If the Care plan includes medication, it is important to measure how the plan moves the patient from assessment to action (see KPI 9—comprehensive care plan acceptance rate and KPI 10—time to medication initiation).

The second thing it detects is whether anyone has built a plan. A patient who starts medication without a Care plan is a patient whose clinician wrote a prescription and moved on. The plan is what turns the prescription into a treatment course. These two metrics measure the first 30 days. Did the patient take the first dose of a recommended medication? Did the program give them a Care plan? If the answer to either question is no, the program is little more than an e-commerce platform masquerading as a medical practice.

KPI 09 OF 50

COMPONENT	LENS	TIER
CARE	**PROGRAM STEWARDSHIP**	**EXPERIENCE**

KPI **COMPREHENSIVE CARE PLAN ACCEPTANCE RATE**

The share of patients who accept a documented, clinician-countersigned comprehensive Care plan within 30 days of enrollment.

MEASURES	Patients with a signed Care plan in the record within 30 days, divided by all enrolled patients in the monthly cohort. The plan addresses pharmacotherapy titration, nutrition, movement, sleep, and coordination of comorbidities. It is co-built with the patient, not handed to them.
SIGNAL	A high rate means patients leave the first month with a clinical roadmap they helped build. A low rate means the program started medication without the scaffolding that makes the medication work.
TIMEFRAME	Day 0 to Day 30 from enrollment, reported by monthly cohort.

KPI 10 OF 50

COMPONENT	LENS	TIER
CARE	**PATIENT BEHAVIOR**	**EXPERIENCE**

KPI **TIME TO MEDICATION INITIATION**

The median number of days between prescription issuance and patient-confirmed first dose.

MEASURES	Days from prescription date to patient-confirmed first dose. Fill data alone is insufficient; confirmation of the injection itself is required. The 90th percentile is tracked alongside the median as the tail indicator. This does not reward rushing to pharmacotherapy immediately on enrollment. For some, this is good Care. For others, a delay is better.
SIGNAL	A short, stable median means the Care layer is closing the gap between prescription and action. A long or lengthening median means patients are missing implementation support. Discovering the barrier to action should be led by Care.
TIMEFRAME	Reported monthly on the cohort of patients prescribed that month.

GOOD CARE HANDLES COMPLEXITY

If I were looking at Wayne's case and faced with the same question (*should he increase his semaglutide to 1.7 mg?*), I would have many questions. In practice, a strong clinical record, driven by Wayne's engagement with the other components and his past check-ins, would surface these answers for me at a glance. I would corroborate during a one-to-one visit and help him decide what to do.

How much weight has he lost, and when? Thirty-five pounds in four months is nearly 10% of his starting weight. But was the loss front-loaded in the first six weeks, or steady across 16? Has he truly plateaued, or is the scale simply stalling for three weeks? Three weeks is not always a plateau. Six weeks, though, probably is.

What is happening with his blood pressure? His cardiology note says "stable," but that was written in the cardiologist's office in the late afternoon. Cardiologists have a way of raising their patients' blood pressures by their mere presence. Also, if Wayne had a salty lunch, then the office measure may mislead us. I want his weekly home measures, taken in the morning before he takes his medications and has a coffee. My clinical software should surface this, too. If his home readings are around 128/80 mmHg while sitting and he is not dizzy when standing, we have room to maneuver. He is very tall, and there is a lot of gravity to contend with when he goes from lying down to standing up. If they are closer to 118/78 mmHg and he reports occasional lightheadedness, a higher dose of semaglutide may reduce his water and food intake, thereby lowering his blood pressure. This could cause falls or leave him very tired. I would recommend preemptively lowering his blood pressure medication in the latter case but holding steady in the former.

Wayne's LDL cholesterol (sometimes called *bad* cholesterol) is 145 mg/dL (3.75 mmol/L) while on a statin. His cardiologist wants it below 100 mg/dL (2.6 mmol/L). Semaglutide helps with LDL, but the effect is stronger at higher doses. If he increases his semaglutide and statin at the same time and he feels terrible, we will have to troubleshoot which medication caused which symptom. Whichever decision is made, a quick note to his cardiologist is a good idea. The system should generate this for me in a few seconds and send it off automatically.

Is he eating enough food? I would like to know how many calories below his daily needs he is getting. The Connection component of the Canopy provides this information in real time (which will be covered in more detail in Chapter 16). If Wayne is eating about the same amount his body needs and is struggling to manage cravings after dinner, he would benefit from a higher dose. If he is already eating 1,000 fewer calories than his daily requirement with little effort, he does not need a higher dose. He may actually be eating too little, causing his metabolism to downshift. This is one of the counter-regulatory mechanisms the body utilizes to protect against weight loss, because weight loss signals danger to our primitive brains. If he eats a little bit more—ideally only 500 calories below his daily requirement—he may feel even better, and his metabolism would rise accordingly. He may find more motivation to move and note improvements in his mood. At 1 mg of semaglutide, I don't want to lower his dose and lose the pan-metabolic benefits of the medication, but he may need to eat a little bit more to keep his weight loss moving.

This part of the clinical decision making often disorients patients. Eat more? To lose weight? To an extent, yes. The rise of diet culture has indoctrinated whole generations into believing they need to be dramatically underfed in order to lose weight. They all point to past experiences with commercial diets where they "succeeded." Patients often feel the need to actively restrict calories when on obesity medications because they're used to their lives being broken into phases: on track and off track. When they are on track, they follow the *diet* and eat *perfectly*. In the modern era, they also associate these turns with taking their medication and eating much less food, even if it takes superhuman effort. Off track is associated with not taking medication and eating whatever works. This polarization is not helpful for patients and can result in big fueling swings. Wayne's basal metabolic rate is well over 2,000 calories. If he is eating 1,200 calories and feels fine, he will start losing muscle as well as fat, and the fatigue will catch up with him within a month.

Is he eating enough protein? The evidence supports 1.2–1.6 grams per kilogram of lean mass for patients on these medications.[4] Most patients do not hit that without deliberate effort. If Wayne is eating 60 grams of protein a day and losing five pounds a month, he cannot protect his lean mass. I need to know where his food intake stands before I add more appetite suppression.

How is his sleep? Poor sleep drives insulin resistance, which blunts the medication's effect. How is his mood? Wayne already has challenges with executive function and mood regulation. Rapid weight loss without adequate nutrition can worsen both. Is he constipated? Constipation is common with these medications, and escalating the dose will make it worse. Does the injection-day nausea affect his eating, or is it just transient discomfort? Nausea that causes meal-skipping on a GLP-1 creates a vicious cycle: less food, more nausea, less food, etc.

Would he prefer an intermediate step? The injection pens can dispense in small increments. Wayne could technically give himself a dose that is between 1 mg and 1.7 mg, but it is off-label and high-risk for dosing error, especially in someone with poor vision or dexterity. But some patients do better adjusting the dose to 1.25 mg for a month before jumping to 1.7 mg. Others prefer or need simplicity.

Care infrastructure that enables a clinical team to perform expert analysis of many variables under protocols, using AI-augmented workflows, is what makes obesity medicine possible at scale, given the relatively few specialists available. It also demonstrates that providing quality care to people with obesity is about far more than medication.

The Obesity Medicine Education Collaborative defines 32 core competencies for obesity medicine practice, including pharmacotherapy selection, titration protocols, and comorbidity coordination.[5] Those competencies do not require a specialist for every encounter. A nurse practitioner or pharmacist, operating under a protocol authored by a specialist team, can scale. The specialist serves as the escalation tier, handling complex cases, coordinating across specialties, and making decisions that fall outside the protocol. This limited attention can go to the patients who need it most. A patient whose trajectory fits the protocol will receive the protocol's benefit without the wait.

This is the Livongo model mentioned in Chapter 7: attention routed by data rather than by appointment slot. A stable patient with no side effects does not need a synchronous visit with a physician. A patient whose weight has stalled for six weeks or whose blood pressure has dropped by 20 points needs expert clinical attention now, not at the next scheduled appointment.

The Institute for Clinical and Economic Review's cost-effectiveness models for obesity pharmacotherapy are sensitive to exactly these delivery ratios.[6] When the models assume physician-only delivery, cost per quality-adjusted life-year exceeds willingness-to-pay thresholds. When they assume protocol-governed task shifting with specialist oversight, it falls below the threshold. The difference is not the cost of the medication. It is about the organization and execution of Care.

CARE PLANS LIVE

After the first month, Care shifts from building the plan to keeping it relevant to a changing patient. Two KPIs measure Care engagement for months 2 through 12 (see KPI 11—pharmacotherapy cessation rate and KPI 12—care plan update acceptance rate).

When Care plans are reviewed quarterly, side effects are caught early, doses are adjusted before tolerance fails, and patients stay on medication because someone is actively managing the treatment course. Rodriguez and colleagues found the highest discontinuation risk in months 2 through 6, with a secondary peak in months 10 through 12.[7] About half of these were driven by Cost and Coverage.[8] We need to remember that Cost is about price and perceived value. If a patient is paying a high cost for something that they do not understand, do not feel is working, and makes them feel terrible, then there is no Cost low enough to keep them on medication. The other five components of transformation infrastructure help patients realize value for price. The other leading reason for discontinuation in the first year is side effects. An expert obesity practice has no trouble handling side effects. There are hundreds of strategies we can use to support a patient through these difficult

KPI 11 OF 50

COMPONENT	LENS	TIER
CARE	**PATIENT BEHAVIOR**	**ENGAGEMENT**

KPI **PHARMACOTHERAPY CESSATION RATE**

The share of pharmacotherapy-enrolled patients who stop medication between months 2 and 12 (excluding clinically-indicated de-prescription).

MEASURES

Patients who stop obesity medication, divided by all patients taking obesity medication in the cohort. Cessation is defined as a prescription lapse of 14 days beyond the end of known supply or a patient-reported discontinuation. Patients who unenroll from the entire program should be excluded from the stop group and the entire cohort, as they may be transferring to another practice. The cessation rate is susceptible to data lag in programs where the pharmacy is not directly integrated.

SIGNAL

A low and stable rate means the Care layer is absorbing side effects, adjusting doses, and matching complexity to the patient's life. A rising rate, or a rate concentrated in a particular phase, tells the program where Care is breaking down.

TIMEFRAME

Measured on each monthly enrollment cohort across months 2 through 12; reported as a rolling 12-month cessation curve.

KPI 12 OF 50

COMPONENT	LENS	TIER
CARE	**PROGRAM STEWARDSHIP**	**ENGAGEMENT**

KPI **CARE PLAN UPDATE ACCEPTANCE RATE**

The share of patients whose Care plan is reviewed and updated during months 2 through 12, with the update acknowledged by the patient.

MEASURES	Patients with at least one documented Care plan update accepted during months 2 through 12, divided by all enrolled patients at that time. An update reviews health status, titration, tolerance, behavioral goals, and comorbidity status, with patient acknowledgment on record.
SIGNAL	A high rate means the plan is a living document and the patient is inside the loop.
TIMEFRAME	Measured monthly on the cohort of patients in months two through 12 of treatment.

times. A Care plan can adjust automatically if the system is listening for the right signals at the right time.

Sarah's Question

Sarah comes in at month 3 to request a dose increase. She has been on Wegovy—1 mg of semaglutide—weekly since returning to treatment through her new employer's coverage, and her weight loss has slowed.

Before I discuss the dose, I ask about her sleep. She pauses. She has not been sleeping well. She jolts awake at three o'clock in the morning, and she lies awake for an hour before drifting off again. She has no idea why this keeps happening, and she is exhausted. She keeps skipping her personal trainer sessions because she cannot muster the energy to lift weights.

An expert Care layer recognizes that Sarah is experiencing perimenopausal sleep disturbances. It will get worse before it gets better. No amount of Wegovy will do for Sarah what her ovaries have been doing for decades: sending estrogen and progesterone into circulation to support every other organ in her body.

Poor sleep drives insulin resistance and dysregulates appetite and mood. Weight loss is really difficult under these conditions. Sarah's plateau is not a medication problem. It is a hormone-driven sleep disturbance and, with it, comes a basket of other Care considerations connected to her stage of life. Her libido, ability to think, stress tolerance, and menstrual experience may all be off kilter. Good Care for obesity, in Sarah's context, is good women's health. Her Care plan should be updated to include evaluation for perimenopause and personalized consideration of menopausal hormone therapy. This could be by referral or in-house menopause expertise.

If the Care component does not recognize a new comorbidity and instead increases Wegovy to 1.7 mg per week, Sarah may lose a little more weight, but she will plateau again and continue to feel terrible. She will ask for another dose increase, assuming that if she could just lose more weight, then she would feel better, and the cycle continues. The monocropper's protocol suggests a switch to tirzepatide, but that doesn't work either. Soon, she abandons the program and the treatment together. All because Care was not done well.

I remind Sarah of what I told her in the beginning: faster, higher, and stronger is not the path to sustainable weight management. And then we work on how to get her sleeping through the night.

CARE TRANSFORMS

Care should also be measured by patient outcomes. As a component of transformation infrastructure, Care includes four outcome KPIs drawn from the International Consortium for Health Outcomes Measurement Adult Obesity Standard Set.[9] (See KPI 13—HBA1C change, KPI 14—blood pressure change, KPI 15—lipid panel change, and KPI 16—musculoskeletal pain.) Care carries more outcome KPIs than any other component because its work should most directly produce measurable metabolic and functional change. Let's look at Wayne's transformation.

Wayne's A1c was 6.3% when he restarted treatment. It is now 5.9%. The goal is 5.7%. He is not there yet, but he is moving in the right direction, and he is motivated. He eats three good-sized meals per day and is hungry in the morning. His weight loss has been evenly distributed throughout the treatment period. He has daily bowel movements without straining. He had mild nausea on the first day of treatment, but otherwise feels his side effects do not bother him. He should do well at 1.7 mg.

Wayne's systolic blood pressure is 128 mmHg. His cardiologist is satisfied with that number. What I am watching for is the drop that will come when he loses another 20 pounds. If his average systolic pressure falls below 120, we need to reduce one of his blood pressure medications. If we do not, he will get lightheaded and may attribute his symptoms to the semaglutide itself. In the worst (but totally foreseeable) case, he falls, hits his head, ends up in the hospital with a subdural hematoma, takes months to recover, and has to sell his business—he is never the same.

Wayne's LDL is above target, as are his triglycerides. Semaglutide will help with both, but the effect depends on the dose and weight loss. The Care layer keeps the obesity medicine team and the cardiologist in the same conversation about whether to adjust the statin as the lipids respond.

Wayne finds it a little easier to get into and out of his car now, and his knees feel better. He is more agile and comfortable as each day goes by. This makes it easier for him to enjoy his work and his life.

KPI 13 OF 50

COMPONENT	LENS	TIER
CARE	**OUTCOME**	**OUTCOME**

KPI **HBA1C CHANGE**

Change in glycated hemoglobin (HbA1c) in patients with diabetes and, separately, with prediabetes, measured at baseline and six-month intervals.

MEASURES	Mean change in A1c percentage points at 6 and 12 months, by HbA1c starting cohort.
TIMEFRAME	Measured at 0, 6, and 12 months from baseline, reported as cohort mean change.

KPI 14 OF 50

COMPONENT	LENS	TIER
CARE	**OUTCOME**	**OUTCOME**

KPI **BLOOD PRESSURE CHANGE**

Change in systolic and diastolic blood pressure for patients with hypertension, measured at baseline, 3, 6, and 12 months.

MEASURES	Mean change in mmHg and share of patients reaching target. Tracks antihypertensive dose adjustments in Care plan alongside weight trajectory.
TIMEFRAME	Measured at 0, 3, 6, and 12 months from baseline, reported as cohort mean change.

KPI 15 OF 50

COMPONENT	LENS	TIER
CARE	**OUTCOME**	**OUTCOME**

KPI **LIPID PANEL CHANGE**

Change in LDL, HDL, and triglycerides for patients with dyslipidemia, measured at baseline and annually.

MEASURES	Mean change per test and share of patients reaching LDL target. Tracks statin dose adjustments in Care plan alongside weight trajectory.
TIMEFRAME	Measured at baseline and annually, reported as cohort mean change.

KPI 16 OF 50

COMPONENT	LENS	TIER
CARE	**OUTCOME**	**OUTCOME**

KPI **MUSCULOSKELETAL PAIN**

Patient-reported pain measured by the EQ-5D-5L pain/discomfort score (1 to 5) at baseline and at 6 and 12 months.

MEASURES	Change in pain dimension score (1 to 5). The EQ-5D-5L captures pain on a single pain/discomfort dimension scored one through five. Reported as mean change.
TIMEFRAME	Measured at baseline, 6, and 12 months, reported as cohort mean change.

CARE REQUIRES LEARNING

Sarah sends me a link to a podcast on perimenopause in her patient portal. "I know you were saying something like this in our visit, but it was just so helpful to hear it again from a different perspective," she wrote. Patients sometimes worry that I will be offended if they do their own research. Honestly, it is quite the opposite.

Care can create the conditions for transformation, but it cannot, alone, produce a durable understanding. Curriculum is the next component, and it can have an outsized impact on transformation. Chapter 13 is about what a real curriculum looks like and how to measure it.

Sarah is right. I can't teach her everything she needs to know about her body in every single moment of the day. She needs to know her own operating system. She needs a quality education, designed for adults and for the modern era. Because learning, especially about what she needs in order to heal, is transformation.

ENDNOTES

1. "ABOM Announces October '25 Test Results—American Board of Obesity Medicine," American Board of Obesity Medicine, December 11, 2025, https://www.abom.org/abom-announces-october-25-test-results-2/.
2. Blue Health Intelligence, *Real-World Trends in GLP-1 Treatment Persistence and Prescribing for Weight Management* (Blue Health Intelligence, 2024); Jason M. Samuels et al., "Real-World Titration, Persistence & Weight Loss of Semaglutide and Tirzepatide in an Academic Obesity Clinic," *Diabetes, Obesity and Metabolism* 27, no. 11 (2025): 6200–209, https://doi.org/10.1111/dom.70004.
3. Blue Health Intelligence, *Real-World Trends in GLP-1 Treatment Persistence and Prescribing for Weight Management.*
4. Dariush Mozaffarian et al., "Nutritional Priorities to Support GLP-1 Therapy for Obesity: A Joint Advisory from the American College of Lifestyle Medicine, the American Society for Nutrition, the Obesity Medicine Association, and The Obesity Society," *Obesity* 33, no. 8 (2025): 1475–503, https://doi.org/10.1002/oby.24336.
5. Robert F. Kushner et al., "Development of Obesity Competencies for Medical Education: A Report from the Obesity Medicine Education Collaborative," *Obesity* 27, no. 7 (2019): 1063–67, https://doi.org/10.1002/oby.22471.
6. Grace A. Lin et al., *Semaglutide and Tirzepatide for Obesity: Effectiveness and Value* (Institute for Clinical and Economic Review, 2025).
7. Patricia J. Rodriguez et al., "Discontinuation and Reinitiation of Dual-Labeled GLP-1 Receptor Agonists Among U.S. Adults With Overweight or Obesity," *JAMA Network Open* 8, no. 1 (2025): e2457349, https://doi.org/10.1001/jamanetworkopen.2024.57349.
8. Hamlet Gasoyan et al., "Reasons for Discontinuation of Obesity Pharmacotherapy with Semaglutide or Tirzepatide in Clinical Practice," *Obesity* 33, no. 12 (2025): 2296–303, https://doi.org/10.1002/oby.70058.
9. Teferi Mekonnen et al., "Development of a Core Patient-Centred Outcome Set for Adults Living with Obesity: A Modified Delphi-Based International Consensus," *eClinicalMedicine* 87 (September 2025), https://doi.org/10.1016/j.eclinm.2025.103422.

CHAPTER 13

CURRICULUM IN THE CANOPY

Wayne agreed to an increased dose of Wegovy at his last visit. His medication arrived in the mail, and he started it on time, with Linda's support. He noticed a difference in his appetite right away. He was able to eat, but he just did not want to.

He had a few bites of toast for breakfast and then a half sandwich later in the afternoon. His dinner was balanced but small. He thought this was a good thing. He was full earlier and for longer. He tried his whole life to eat less, and now he finally could. Before the medication, he relied on stomach stretch or on his brain registering that he was stuffed before he could stop eating. He cannot rely on those feelings anymore because they arrive after very little food lands in his gut. He can physically see that he is eating less food, but it still feels like so much more.

At his next check-in, he reports an additional weight loss of 19 lbs—or 6% of his body weight—over four weeks. This should trigger a system-level warning for weight loss above a safe threshold. If this keeps up, Wayne will lose too much muscle to make the weight loss worth it. As he gets older, it is even more important that weight loss be slow enough to allow him to sustain muscle and metabolism, while fat stores decrease.

Instead, his program guide sends him a message: "*Congratulations on your progress, Wayne!*" His buddy Tom told him he looked great at work today. Wayne was really proud of himself. "I can't believe how easy this is," he marveled at Linda. Wayne has no reason to think that 1.7 mg per week is a problem because everyone is celebrating his starvation.

The right Care decision is to throttle back his dose, even if temporarily. But it is not that simple. For the first time in his life, Wayne is experiencing ease with his appetite. This is real relief. At a lower dose, his appetite will be stronger, and Wayne will have to tend to it. Immediately, Wayne will feel like he's backsliding and that the weight will return with a vengeance along with the familiar flood of futility and frustration. In reality, he will keep losing weight at 1 mg per week, manage his appetite, and his effort will pay off. But he won't see that right away. The safe and sustainable downward dose adjustment comes with emotional baggage.

How do we help Wayne understand why he needs more time at 1 mg per week? The Curriculum is the Canopy component that holds learning moments, like the one Wayne needs here. Obesity is a lifelong illness, and it has no cure. People with type 1 diabetes must learn about carbohydrate counting and insulin. The same is true for people with obesity.

"I'm really tired this week," Wayne mentioned to Linda during his third week on 1.7 mg of Wegovy. A few months back, they started taking walks together after dinner, but he could not muster enough energy the last two nights. He was a little bit lightheaded and found himself feeling colder than usual.

He opened a browser and searched, "*How many calories do I actually need?*" A total daily energy expenditure (TDEE) calculator appeared in the results. He punches in his numbers: 64-year-old male, 296 pounds, light activity level. It said he needed to eat 3,339 calories a day to maintain his weight and about 2,700 calories a day to lose a pound per week. Then he opened his food log. He was only eating about 900 calories a day.

He couldn't believe it. Wayne sent a message to the program through the app at 7:14 PM: "*Is my dose too high?*" The next day, he received a basic reply with four article links about *healthy eating on GLP-1 medications*. He read them but was not sure if they applied to him. He would wait until his next check-in to ask again.

HOW WE LEARN

Wayne's message about his dose is a sign of *patient activation*, a term coined by researchers in 2004 to describe how patients can move from being passive recipients of information to active managers of their own disease, and the extent to which that is possible (see Figure 13.1).[1]

The original researchers of this measure found that patients at Level 4 had meaningfully lower rates of emergency department visits and unplanned hospitalizations than those at lower levels across multiple chronic-disease populations.[2] The magnitude depended on the study and the condition, but the direction was consistent. A patient who has taken ownership of their health generates a different utilization profile than one who has not. This is one way in which the patient-care argument and the commercial argument align.

Activation correlates with well-being. UK data show that patients in the highest-activation cohort had 32% fewer emergency department attendances and 38% fewer emergency admissions than those in the lowest.[3] Every Canopy component supports transformation through activation—a process that starts with experience, continues with engagement, and evolves to empowerment. Curriculum provides the underlying knowledge for patients and defines the touchpoints where they can apply it.

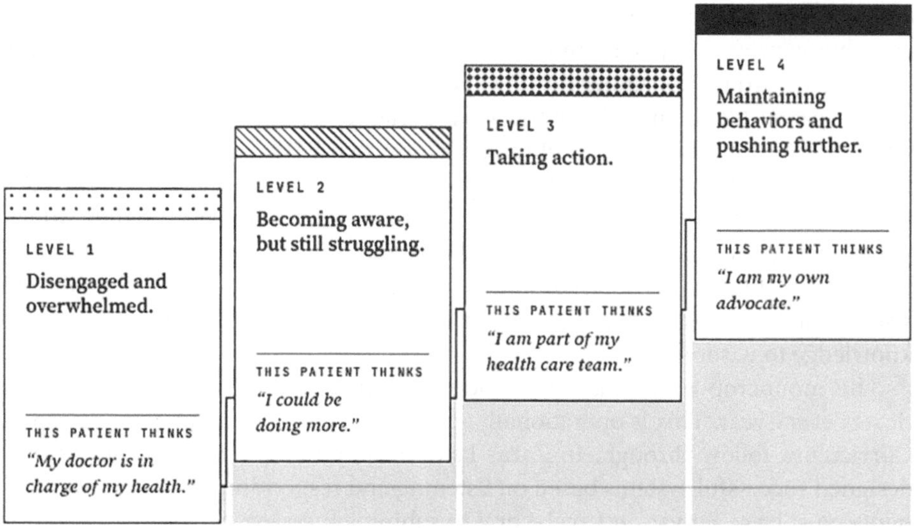

Figure 13.1 Four levels of patient activation. *Source*: NHS England, Personalized Care Group, Patient Activation Team, Module 1: PAM® Implementation Quick Guide, Guidance no. 07888 (NHS England, 2018).

THE STATUS QUO PROBLEM

Patients forget 40% to 80% of medical information within hours of receiving it, and nearly half of what they do retain is recalled incorrectly.[4] This is because adults learn by self-directed discovery and by applying what they know to new situations.[5] The medical appointment is a useless container for adult learning. There is little time for questions; the topics are complex; no one speaks Latin anymore; no two patients have the same baseline knowledge; and nearly all of them have already read something wrong on the internet. Patients are emotional and vulnerable. Clinicians may be hungry for food, time, help, and a bathroom break. Learning inside the *business-as-usual* health care system is an impossible task for everyone involved.

In disrupting the status quo of how we access health care, digital health platforms inadvertently collapsed the old division between traditional health care and the consumer-focused wellness world. Traditional health care relied on *doctors' orders* and patient compliance. The wellness industry leverages consumers' need for choice, identity, and discovery—the keys to adult learning. The monocroppers want the best of both worlds and the hard responsibilities of neither. They want the regulatory moats and the captive patients of the medical system. And they want the unfettered speed, volume, and revenue of the supplement, diet, and lifestyle companies. Yet they filter out patients and ailments that come with complexities and emergencies. They self-commodified instead of innovating toward a unifying higher standard for consumer health experiences.

Companies like Hims & Hers and WW Clinic (formerly WeightWatchers) have knowledge materials—content libraries, blog posts, FAQs, and emails—but stop there. In his 2026 book, *The Transformation Economy*, Joseph Pine calls knowledge the means to which the end is wisdom.[6] Most activations fail because they stop at knowledge and do not follow through to wisdom. One of my patients, Jane, who was instrumental in this book coming to life, says that wisdom is like "metabolized knowledge." Everyone has a different rate for metabolizing food to fuel, but also knowledge to wisdom.

The monocrop programs boast about handling millions of patient support tickets every year. This is operationally impressive, but there is an obvious gap in Curriculum follow-through. In Zara's listen-respond loop from Chapter 8, they designed successful systems based on listening and responding, over and over. Patients must be at activation Level 3 or 4 to submit a message. Most will not ask for help; they will disengage.

THE CURRICULUM LIVES ON

The Curriculum is not the same as onboarding. Pine specifically warns against fixing structured learning to the earliest parts of a transformation. As body weight fluctuates, three things change for a patient: metabolism, appetite, and perspective. In my practice, I call this The MAP™. Patients need to loop back over the ideas and principles that govern their shifting MAP™ over the span of years, not weeks or months.

In weight loss, the more a patient changes, the more they need to learn. But learning itself creates more change. Curriculum is a lifelong constant and should be designed this way. A patient may find a lesson they read during their first month completely forgettable. The first 30 days are for orientation and making space for being overwhelmed. In months 2 to 12, the Curriculum facilitates engagement. A TDEE calculator available to Wayne within his program would not only provide his fuel numbers but also help him understand why they matter.

A working Curriculum is sequenced and evaluated teaching that is delivered professionally, with measured outcomes (see KPI 17—curriculum activation rate). It standardizes content while personalizing the learning path. It relies on teachers who are not always clinicians, including peers. And it extends through the patient's entire chronic disease arc, not just the period of acute weight change.

The sooner a patient activates their learning, the better (see KPI 18—personalized starting unit assignment rate). Activation leads to better patient outcomes

KPI 17 OF 50

COMPONENT	LENS	TIER
CURRICULUM	**PATIENT BEHAVIOR**	**EXPERIENCE**

KPI **CURRICULUM ACTIVATION RATE**

The percentage of patients who, within 30 days of enrollment, complete at least one self-initiated action connected to a curriculum element.

MEASURES	Patient-initiated action occurring at least 60 minutes after any system prompt and containing substantive patient-specific input.
SIGNAL	Low values suggest the curriculum is not reaching patients in the first month. High values indicate the program produced an early patient-led behavior.
TIMEFRAME	30 days from enrollment. Reported monthly across rolling cohorts.

KPI 18 OF 50

COMPONENT	LENS	TIER
CURRICULUM	**PROGRAM STEWARDSHIP**	**EXPERIENCE**

KPI **PERSONALIZED STARTING UNIT ASSIGNMENT RATE**

The percentage of enrolled patients assigned an initial curriculum experience within 30 days, based on at least three documented signals including age, comorbidity status, and one preference or context signal.

MEASURES	Whether the first learning experience is partially segmented and personalized.
SIGNAL	Low values indicate curriculum is largely raw content. High values indicate programmatic flexibility and responsiveness.
TIMEFRAME	30 days from enrollment.

and, in health, as in investing, these will compound over time.[7] But different people need to understand different things, especially early on. A 25-year-old graduate student who suddenly gained 50 pounds on antipsychotic medication has a different starting point than a 55-year-old who has lost and gained the same 100 pounds four times.

This metric tracks whether the program can create useful learning moments for patients before it has had time to get to know them well. Three basic demographic intake signals will not produce a custom Curriculum, but they will produce a starting unit that is closer to the patient than a generic welcome flow. This is early personalization at work.

THE RESTRICTION ERA IS OVER

Sarah has counted calories in everything she has eaten for over 20 years. Sometimes this is effective for sustaining weight loss, but oftentimes it is not (see Figure 13.2). She started dieting earnestly during college. She joined formal programs, all of which told her that effort creates outcome and restriction is reward. And now she has to shake it all off so that she can safely manage the chronic disease that is obesity. For Sarah, the Curriculum challenge is not learning new information. It is unlearning the operating system that twenty years of diet culture installed.

If the Curriculum component does not reveal this and replace it, Sarah will use the medication to perform the diets she knows so well. The Curriculum must teach and welcome nourishment. This is going to look different for different groups of patients, in different countries, and at different life stages. But nourishment is the critical priority for the future of obesity medicine.

The urgency of learning and unlearning is only increasing. Retatrutide and CagriSema are in late-stage trials. These medications are expected to be very powerful. Ironically, the more effective the medication, the more emphasis is needed on nourishment. The more powerful the appetite suppression, the more Sarah needs a Curriculum that gives her permission to nourish, after decades of restriction.

The challenge is that a new meal plan does not do this. Information about protein targets and micronutrient adequacy does not do this. Sarah has to encounter the evidence that the restriction failed her systemically, not personally. She has to reach her own conclusion. The Curriculum's job is to build the conditions for that encounter, not to hand her a corrected belief.

The Curriculum has to address patients' beliefs about whether treatment is necessary and worth the difficulty. It must also attune to the patient's actual capacity to learn.[8] Wayne understands why he takes semaglutide and has accepted the tradeoffs. But he does not know how to titrate his dose or food to his appetite. He also

Some companies make claims that do not line up with the scientific evidence on weight loss.

Noom markets a *"Taper-Off Guarantee."* It promises that behavioral coaching can transition patients off GLP-1 medications while they keep the weight loss. Both companies pitch this to payers as cost savings: invest in our behavioral platform, and you can stop paying for expensive medications.

The weight-regain data after medication discontinuation contradict these claims. When patients stop GLP-1 treatment, their appetite returns. The metabolic changes that made weight loss so hard before treatment have not disappeared. They were suppressed. Remove the suppression, and the biological pressure reasserts itself. Nearly every patient who loses weight will regain it without intervention.

The off-ramp pitch recreates the dieting model, just with medications as a temporary bridge. It assumes the problem is behavioral: teach people the right habits, and the medication becomes unnecessary. But obesity is a chronic disease with biological drivers. Treating it as a behavioral problem that medications can temporarily solve is the same framework that produced 90 years of failed dieting and the current obesity epidemic.

Figure 13.2 The off-ramp does not exist.

Source: Noom, "Noom Introduces Industry-First $129 Compounded GLP-1 with a Taper-Off Guarantee, Offering a Sustainable Approach to Long-Term Weight Loss," In the News, December 5, 2025, https://www.noom.com/in-the-news/glp-1rx/.

does not recognize that his metabolism can change in response to what he eats; therefore, he needs help grasping the long-term implications. Sarah is working to understand that she can feed herself well and still lose weight—and then maintain it. She has never before existed in a world where she could do both over the long term (see Figure 13.3).

After the first month, the Curriculum's role shifts to what Lorig and Holman call *self-tailoring*.[9] Self-tailoring is the deepest behavioral signature of learning on the road to transformation. A self-tailoring patient does not need to be told what to do. They just need the program to stay beside them while they figure it out (see KPI 19—unit progression rate).

A curriculum interaction qualifies as an applied learning touchpoint when it includes *both*:

(a) educational content addressing a relevant topic, and

(b) a way to apply or practice with the new content within 30 minutes.

+ **A nutrition lesson paired with an integrated meal-logging tool qualifies, as does a coaching session on goal-setting.**
- **An emailed article that points the patient to an external food-logging app does not.**

Figure 13.3 Applied learning touchpoints.

The Curriculum should clarify where each patient is at the beginning and help them progress toward transformation. After the first month, the Curriculum should help patients understand, grow, and change (see KPI 20—adaptive progression rate). What matters is the distance traveled for each patient, not an arbitrary set of goalposts applied uniformly to every patient. Growth is growth. A Canopy program is one where patients want to engage, creating the conditions for the third tier of transformation—empowerment. Well-designed digital health experiences leverage the arc of transformation to help patients create more health for themselves.[10]

Adaptive progression at any meaningful scale requires automation, or what is known in digital health as just-in-time adaptive interventions (JITAI).[11] With these, a patient's behavior inside the Curriculum signals readiness to adapt. That signal requires the program to hear the signal, predict the patient's next needs, and respond with an adapted Curriculum experience.

Each adaptive event also raises the patient's investment in the program through the *endowment effect*: people value what they already have, and the longer they have held a service relationship, the higher the cost of leaving it.[12] A patient at month 8 has eight months of Curriculum progress, coaching notes, body-composition trends, and community relationships sitting inside the program. It cannot simply be ported outside of the Canopy because it was co-created by the patient and the Canopy's transformation infrastructure. Here, the retention argument and the transformation argument are one and the same.

KPI 19 OF 50

COMPONENT	LENS	TIER
CURRICULUM	**PATIENT BEHAVIOR**	**ENGAGEMENT**

KPI **UNIT PROGRESSION RATE**

The percentage of active patients per month who actively apply learning inside a curriculum experience and advance to the next curriculum experience.

MEASURES	Whether the curriculum sustains engagement into the next learning experience.
SIGNAL	Progression rising from month two through month seven or eight indicates the curriculum is progressing evenly as patients learn. Flat progression indicates barriers to engagement and activation are present.
TIMEFRAME	Monthly, months two through 12.

KPI 20 OF 50

COMPONENT	LENS	TIER
CURRICULUM	**PROGRAM STEWARDSHIP**	**ENGAGEMENT**

KPI **ADAPTIVE PROGRESSION RATE**

The percentage of active patients whose curriculum experience is adapted (up or down or across) in a given month based on documented (dis)engagement signals.

MEASURES	The listen-respond-predict-listen loop inside Curriculum.
SIGNAL	A 2:1 or 3:1 ratio of adjusted curriculum to non-adjusted curriculum will give personalized depth.
TIMEFRAME	Monthly.

ENDNOTES

1. Judith H. Hibbard and Jessica Greene, "What the Evidence Shows About Patient Activation: Better Health Outcomes and Care Experiences; Fewer Data on Costs," *Health Affairs* (Project Hope) 32, no. 2 (2013): 207–14, https://doi.org/10.1377/hlthaff.2012.1061.
2. Hibbard and Greene, "What the Evidence Shows About Patient Activation."
3. Mark Kutner et al., *The Health Literacy of America's Adults: Results from the 2003 National Assessment of Adult Literacy*, NCES 2006-483 (National Center for Education Statistics, U.S. Department of Education, 2006).
4. Roy P. C. Kessels, "Patients' Memory for Medical Information," *Journal of the Royal Society of Medicine* 96, no. 5 (2003): 219–22, https://doi.org/10.1258/jrsm.96.5.219.
5. Malcolm S. Knowles et al., *The Adult Learner: The Definitive Classic in Adult Education and Human Resource Development*, 8th ed. (Routledge, 2015).
6. Joseph B. Pine, *The Transformation Economy: Guiding Customers to Achieve Their Aspirations* (Harvard Business Review Press, 2026).
7. Jennifer B. Bollyky et al., "Remote Lifestyle Coaching Plus a Connected Glucose Meter with Certified Diabetes Educator Support Improves Glucose and Weight Loss for People with Type 2 Diabetes," *Journal of Diabetes Research* 2018 (May 2018): 3961730, https://doi.org/10.1155/2018/3961730.
8. R. Horne and J. Weinman, "Patients' Beliefs About Prescribed Medicines and Their Role in Adherence to Treatment in Chronic Physical Illness," *Journal of Psychosomatic Research* 47, no. 6 (1999): 555–67, https://doi.org/10.1016/s0022-3999(99)00057-4.
9. Kate R. Lorig and Halsted Holman, "Self-Management Education: History, Definition, Outcomes, and Mechanisms," *Annals of Behavioral Medicine: A Publication of the Society of Behavioral Medicine* 26, no. 1 (2003): 1–7, https://doi.org/10.1207/S15324796ABM2601_01.
10. Michele L. Patel et al., "Self-Monitoring via Digital Health in Weight Loss Interventions: A Systematic Review Among Adults with Overweight or Obesity," *Obesity* (Silver Spring, Md.) 29, no. 3 (2021): 478–99, https://doi.org/10.1002/oby.23088.
11. Inbal Nahum-Shani et al., "Just-in-Time Adaptive Interventions (JITAIs) in Mobile Health: Key Components and Design Principles for Ongoing Health Behavior Support," *Annals of Behavioral Medicine: A Publication of the Society of Behavioral Medicine* 52, no. 6 (2018): 446–62, https://doi.org/10.1007/s12160-016-9830-8.
12. Richard Thaler, "Toward a Positive Theory of Consumer Choice," *Journal of Economic Behavior & Organization* 1, no. 1 (1980): 39–60, https://doi.org/10.1016/0167-2681(80)90051-7; Daniel Kahneman et al., "Anomalies: The Endowment Effect, Loss Aversion, and Status Quo Bias," *Journal of Economic Perspectives* 5, no. 1 (1991): 193–206, https://doi.org/10.1257/jep.5.1.193.

CHAPTER 14

COACH IN THE CANOPY

Wayne is rummaging through the cupboards. It is a Tuesday afternoon, two weeks after the clinical team reduced his semaglutide dosage back down to 1 mg. The kitchen smells faintly of coffee and Linda's fresh basil. He pulls out a sleeve of crackers, then a handful of almonds, then puts both back. He is hunting for something that will raise his energy level quickly. He does not know what.

Linda is at the counter sorting mail. She watches him for a moment. She has not seen him do this in months. The food-seeking, the rummaging, the way his attention narrows around a snack in the middle of the afternoon. It is something he has done since long before they were married, and it stopped only when his appetite diminished at 1.7 mg. Now, two weeks back at the lower dose, it is back.

"Wayne," she says mildly, "Did you eat lunch?"

He stops with his hand on the cupboard door. He thinks about the morning. The drive into work and the back-to-back meetings. Then he remembers the container of leftover chicken still in the fridge at his office, where he set it down at 11:30 and never picked it up again. He turns toward Linda.

"No, I forgot," he says. "And now my appetite is up because my weight is down and my dose is down. I'm hunting for something that's going to give me fuel quickly."

Linda does not say it for him. She does not tell him "I told you so," or sigh, or solve it for him. She listens, the way she has been listening for thirty years, and when he pauses, she asks, "What do you want to do about it?" This is coaching.

BRIDGING THE KNOW-DO GAP

Wayne is developing the working language for his own appetite patterns, his post-meal sleepiness, and the way an unfed afternoon hijacks his evening. The Curriculum work he has done over the last seven months means he can describe it all. What he is still working on is the bridge between knowing it and acting on it.

Coach is the trunk of the Canopy that turns information into behavior, education into practice, and motivation into activation. Curriculum teaches the patient what they need to know. Coach helps the patient act on what they have learned.

Self-efficacy is a patient's belief that they can do something to achieve the results they want.[1] Self-efficacy shows up in the actions the patient chooses, the effort put into those actions, and how long they persist when things feel like they aren't working. Patients who are very aware and well-resourced say they want to take action on their health all the time, but often do not follow through. They have endless self-efficacy in every part of their lives, but healthy behaviors seem to be out of reach for so many. That is because self-efficacy alone is not enough.

Follow-through requires a patient to seriously want the result for themselves. This is one of the most important ideas from the self-determination theory, which finds that people need autonomy to decide what matters to them and, when they have it, their motivation sticks.[2] The Patient Activation Measure® levels introduced in Chapter 13 show us the same arc, from the patient who says "my doctor is in charge of my health" to the patient who says "I am my own advocate."[3] What all three frameworks describe is a shift *inside* the patient. Coach is the relational infrastructure that can produce that shift.

Robot versus Human Coaching

Most of the literature on how to blend automated and human coaching dates back to the pre-AI era. In the AI-plus-GLP-1 era, we have little nonindustry-funded research to guide the best Coach configurations, but we have also blown the roof off the *art of the possible*. The evidence to date is that human contact, in any modality with substantive engagement, outperforms fully automated systems, and the most durable models augment the human with technology rather than replacing the human. Two examples from recent evidence stand out:

PREPWELL is a digital surgical *prehabilitation* program in the United Kingdom that uses digital structured coaching to prepare patients in the weeks leading up to major elective surgery. In a 2022 evaluation, the program tracked Patient Activation Measure® scores at baseline and at eight weeks. Of the patients who scored level one or two at baseline, where patients see the doctor as in charge of their health, 69% had moved to level three or four by week eight, where the patients see themselves as part of the care team and as their own advocates.[4]

Noom began in behavioral weight management and expanded into GLP-1-supported care through 2024 and 2025. In February 2026, Noom published a cohort analysis of more than 14,000 of its GLP-1 patients, scoring coaching engagement by frequency and depth of patient interaction with the coaching team. The top quartile of engaged patients maintained their subscriptions 2.2 times longer than the bottom quartile and renewed at twice the rate. This cohort is the largest published GLP-1-plus-coaching engagement analysis to date.[5]

THE PATIENT'S CHOICE

A real coaching relationship begins with the patient making a choice, however small. And there are no right answers here: chat is not always better than video; AI is not necessarily better than humans, etc. The point is not which modality wins with every patient; the point is that the patient exercised preference. That preference is the smallest possible behavioral marker that the patient is entering a relationship rather than receiving a service. Each program designs Coach configurability based on its model of care, scale, ideal patient, and margin. The program crafts the dimensions of choice and how it is presented at enrollment. These early design choices create the behaviors of transformation (see KPI 21—coach experience selection rate and KPI 22—coach experience configurability).

KPI 21 OF 50

COMPONENT	LENS	TIER
COACH	**PATIENT BEHAVIOR**	**EXPERIENCE**

KPI **COACH EXPERIENCE SELECTION RATE**

Percentage of enrolled patients who, within 30 days of enrollment, make an active, documented selection of their coach experience from program-offered options. The selection set is program-defined and may include coach modality (chat, video, group, one-to-one, voice note, asynchronous messaging), coach type (AI avatar, human coach, hybrid), specific coach profile from a menu, session format, or cadence. What is measured is that the patient exercised preference, not which option was chosen.

MEASURES	Whether the patient is entering a coaching relationship (preference exercised) rather than receiving a program feature (default assigned).
SIGNAL	Sub-50 percent indicates either the selection flow is missed at enrollment, the options are not meaningful, or the patient has not yet engaged with the relational layer.
TIMEFRAME	First 30 days from enrollment.

KPI 22 OF 50

COMPONENT	LENS	TIER
COACH	**PROGRAM STEWARDSHIP**	**EXPERIENCE**

KPI **COACH EXPERIENCE CONFIGURABILITY**

Binary score per program. The program scores Yes only if all four conditions are met.

CONDITIONS

(1) At least two distinct dimensions of coaching choice, each with at least two meaningful options.

(2) The dimensions are documented in a published coaching taxonomy.

(3) The selection is actively presented at enrollment as a visible choice.

(4) The selection is captured in the record and is consequential, materially shaping what the patient subsequently experiences.

MEASURES	Whether the program has built the substrate that makes Coach Experience Selection possible.
SIGNAL	Yes or No, audited against the four conditions.
TIMEFRAME	Program-level audit, reported quarterly to capture structural change.

THE PATIENT WHO GOES QUIET

The most clinically meaningful Coach metric is the one that detects when the patient goes quiet. Patients who are doing well self-select toward sharing wins with their Coach. They are also sensitive to what they perceive matters to their Coach. If they feel that gaining weight will disappoint their coach, they may hold back from sharing, even if they need support to understand what happened. Shame holds patients in isolation, unless the system is designed for difficulty.

In the world of modern weight loss, there are always side effects:

- Real or perceived weight plateaus
- Arguments about budgets and food selection
- Difficulty with other medical conditions
- Poor sleep
- Bias
- The re-emergence of difficult emotions that were once managed with eating

A transactional coaching relationship is one in which the patient shares a laundry list of successes and is quietly patted on the back. This kind of relationship will not endure. A transformative coaching relationship understands that the Coach is along for the ride this patient is on, no matter how hard or how easy it is at any given time. Programs must decide what counts as a difficult event and what counts as a substantive coaching response to that event.

The Substantive Response Rule

A program response is substantive when it meets one or more of four elements:

1. Informational content
2. Emotional support
3. Acknowledgment of the patient with specificity—a detail she shared rather than a generic phrase
4. Advocacy content or action

Single-emoji reactions, templated automated messages, tag-only replies, self-referential responses, login events without documented participation, copy-paste resource links without context, and one-line acknowledgments do not count. A reaction emoji is not substantive. "Hang in there" is not substantive. A copy-paste resource link without context is not substantive.

The patient's behavior during difficulty is one signal. What the program builds underneath that signal is another. A coaching layer needs to engage with the difficult moments and also be present for the mundane (see KPI 23—coach engagement during difficulty rate and KPI 24—patient-led agenda continuity).

KPI 23 OF 50

COMPONENT	LENS	TIER
COACH	**PATIENT BEHAVIOR**	**ENGAGEMENT**

KPI **COACH ENGAGEMENT DURING DIFFICULTY RATE**

Percentage of patient-flagged difficulty events per quarter where the patient engaged the coach within 7 days of the event. Difficulty events are program-defined. Coach engagement is substantive participation in any program-defined modality.

MEASURES	Whether the coaching relationship has been established to support difficulty.
SIGNAL	Rising rates trended across quarters indicate the coaching layer is the trusted relational surface for hard moments. Flat or declining rates indicate the coaching relationship is not the place patients go when things are hard.
TIMEFRAME	Quarterly across months two through 12. Reported as rolling rate.

KPI 24 OF 50

COMPONENT	LENS	TIER
COACH	**PROGRAM STEWARDSHIP**	**ENGAGEMENT**

KPI **PATIENT-LED AGENDA CONTINUITY**

Percentage of months during months two through 12 in which a patient maintains an active, patient-led agenda within the program. A patient-led agenda is a program-hosted artifact, a working list or goal set or roadmap, that the patient generates and updates. "Active" requires at least one self-initiated substantive update per month, more than 60 minutes after any related system prompt.

MEASURES	Whether the program has built the substrate for patient-driven agency and kept it alive across the program experience.
SIGNAL	Mature programs see cohort averages climb up and to the right. Flat or declining trajectories indicate the agenda infrastructure is not sticky, or the program is building directive structures that crowd out patient-led work.
TIMEFRAME	Monthly per patient; cohort-averaged; trended across the 12-month arc.

WAYNE'S COACH

When Wayne enrolled, the program presented him with a three-dimensional coaching selection: modality (chat, voice note, or video), type (human coach, AI companion, or hybrid), and cadence (weekly, biweekly, or on-demand). Wayne prefers asynchronous communication. He chose to message with an AI Coach and see a human coach every other week. His selection was routed through the platform's logic, shaping his early experience. He got a message from the program's Coach and started turning his thoughts into words.

Wayne knows to get ahead of difficult events before they become difficult weeks or months. In the kitchen with Linda, Wayne picked up his phone and dictated a message. It felt good to reflect out loud on what he learned from missing his lunch. Linda has been writing in her own notebook for years, but Wayne has not been able to find consistent practice for himself. He finds keeping his patient agenda helpful. The agenda started out as a simple weight loss *to-do* list, but it also helps him stay focused on what he wants for his health. It also helps him keep track of when he needs blood tests and when his appointments are.

Linda is, by nature, a Coach. She is curious. She believes Wayne can do this. She holds him in positive regard when he repeats the pattern he has repeated for thirty years. She does not fix his problems for him but sticks with him as he figures it out. She helps him stay accountable to his own goals. Most patients do not have a *Linda*, but everyone needs a *Coach*.

PROFILE: NYMBLE.HEALTH—CLOSING THE KNOW-DO GAP

Company: nymble health
Founded: April 2024
Country: Canada
Co-Founded by: 2x Health Tech Founder and Family Doctor: Dr. Puneet Seth and Endocrinologist: Dr. Megha Poddar

nymble in My Practice

I use nymble in my practice to support patients between visits and to build the core skills of appetite and weight regulation. As my practice changes, my use of nymble will too. My patients often tell me about new nymble use cases they discovered when troubleshooting an issue. I include this case because it demonstrates how Coach can be operationalized at scale in obesity treatment right now, using existing technology that functions within the constraints of real-world practices.

Wayne and nymble

If Wayne's AI chat support from Chapter 14 had been nymble, his experiences in Chapters 13 and 14 would have been quite different. In Chapter 14, Wayne needed to strategize how to stop missing meals. After realizing he missed lunch again, Wayne would have pulled out his phone, opened nymble, and dictated (see Figure 14.1).

The Behavior Gap

The evidence-based guidelines for obesity treatment are unambiguous. Behavioral therapy is foundational, particularly when pharmacotherapy is introduced. Even though access to GLP-1 medications has expanded, the infrastructure required to support behavior change has not followed.

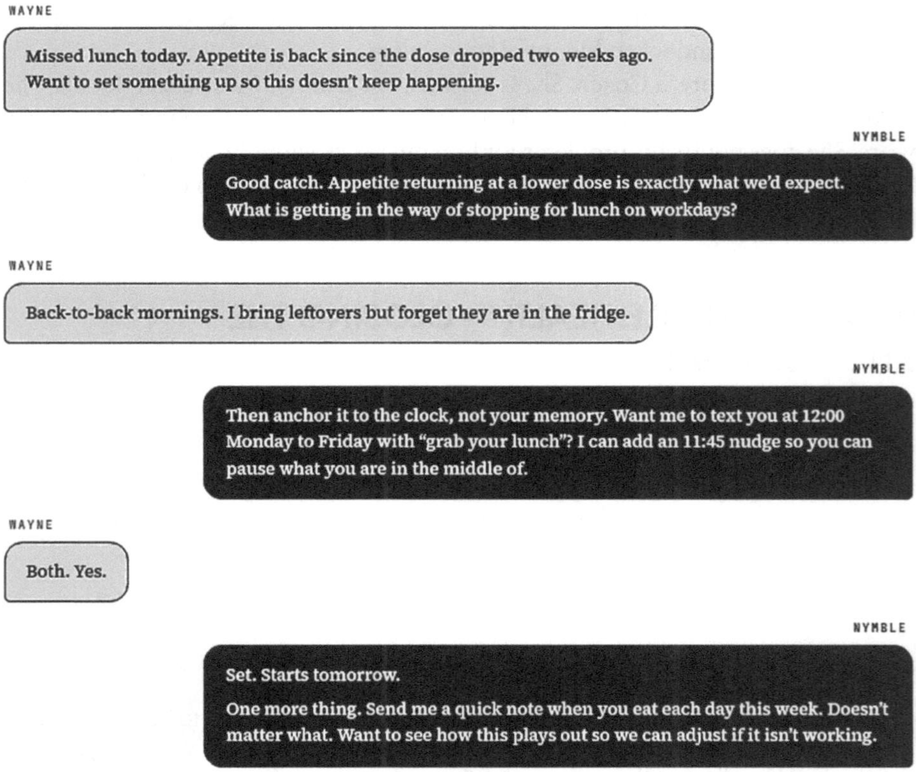

Figure 14.1 Wayne and Coach nymble.

Patients receive expensive medications without continuous behavioral support, then try to navigate side effects, plateaus, and their returning appetites alone for months between clinic visits. Discontinuation rates in the first 12 months exceed 65% in real-world settings. Many patients cannot afford the medications at all. The gap looks different in each cohort: *on medication*, it is the absence of a *guide* between visits; *off medication*, it is the absence of *infrastructure* for sustaining behavior change.

Health systems do not reimburse behavioral support at scale. Most clinicians are not trained to deliver it consistently. Before nymble, the gap was filled with fragments: brief counseling during visits, referral to overburdened dietitians, or consumer apps that exclude older adults, patients with low digital literacy, lower-income patients, and patients who do not speak English.

What nymble Is

nymble is the behavioral infrastructure that makes obesity treatment work at scale. It is a consumer messaging platform delivered through SMS and WhatsApp. There is no app to download, no patient portal to log into, and no synchronous appointment to book. Patients receive proactive education calibrated to their treatment phase; evidence-based responses around the clock with clinical monitoring in the background; configurable reminders; and a proprietary metabolic score, in their preferred language, on the phones they already use.

nymble is available two ways: (1) patients can subscribe directly, with a free starter period followed by a low monthly subscription, or (2) clinics, health systems, and industry partners can license it as customizable infrastructure with a provider portal for data insights.

For clinical partners, nymble reduces the invisible labor of behavioral care and lowers the volume of reactive inbox messages and emergency calls about predictable side effects. The provider portal reveals medical history intake, digital questionnaires, and structured follow-ups. It makes the patient's conversation log available for clinical review before each visit. The platform extends care between appointments without adding to the clinician's day.

For consumers without a clinical relationship, nymble supports behavior change, appetite awareness, and sustainable routines on its own.

From Confusion to Competence

nymble targets the drivers of medication discontinuation that patients can actually control. Its objective is self-efficacy: the patient's confidence that they can take action to achieve the result they want.

Over three to six months, patients build knowledge (*obesity is a chronic disease of appetite regulation; returning hunger signals the need for dose adjustment rather than medication failure*), learn practical skills (*managing nausea, interpreting plateaus without disengaging*), and develop psychological resilience (*hunger is a biological signal, not personal failure*).

When a patient texts "I feel like I'm failing because I'm still hungry sometimes," nymble responds with the actual biology, then asks what is happening in her week that the hunger might be tracking. The shift from confusion and self-blame to context and competence is what supports long-term persistence. The impact is largest in the first six months, when discontinuation risk is highest and behavioral support is most absent.

Implementation at Scale

nymble was built for scale from inception. Deployment requires minimal infrastructure: no app downloads, no mandatory electronic health record integration, and clinician training that often runs under 30 minutes. The platform supports multiple languages and does not rely on synchronous appointments. From signed agreement to live deployment, implementation typically takes two to four weeks. A health system can onboard hundreds or thousands of patients without adding clinical staff.

Unit Economics

Direct-to-consumer pricing runs under $15 per user per month after a free starter period. For organizations and partners, tiered pricing decreases as volume increases. Set that against what nymble offsets:

- **Human-delivered behavioral programs:** $50–$200 per patient per month, capped by clinician availability
- **Avoidable clinic visits:** $150–$300 per reassurance-driven appointment
- **Clinical intake tools:** $150–$300 per month in fees to digital health vendors
- **Lost medication value:** $500–$1,000 per month in wasted pharmacotherapy when patients discontinue prematurely

If nymble prevents one avoidable visit per patient per year, it pays for itself. If it extends medication persistence by three months, the return is substantial, clinically and financially.

The Clinical-Commercial Alignment

What clinicians call nymble: coaching, behavioral support for obesity treatment, clinical infrastructure, medication-adherence counseling, patient education, and engagement.

What pharmaceutical manufacturers, payers, and governments *should* call nymble: the missing layer that determines whether prescribed medications produce real-world results. For health systems, it solves the math of providing continuous, evidence-based support to thousands of patients without hiring hundreds of clinicians. For drugmakers, the persistence layer protects the long arc of a patient's treatment relationship.

Myths and Reality

Three long-held myths about digital behavioral health collapse under the weight of nymble's data.

The first is that digital platforms are not effective. For nymble, the engagement rates at six months are two to three times higher than those of conventional chronic-disease apps. In a clinical pilot, adherence to GLP-1 therapy was 27% higher among patients using nymble than among those receiving standard care. The high engagement at six months reflects the platform working as designed and supporting patients through the phases of treatment and beyond. Sustained engagement rises when patients are met where they already use the service, in their language, with no portal in the way.

The second is that regulatory and clinical complexity are unmanageable barriers to deployment. nymble goes live in two to four weeks under clinician leadership, on existing evidence, using infrastructure the health system already owns. Complexity is a function of the architecture chosen, not of the field.

The third is that digital health tools work only for young, tech-savvy, English-speaking patients. SMS reaches older adults, patients with low digital literacy, and patients who do not speak English—precisely the populations that app-based solutions filter out by design.

> ***"Medications do not fail people. Systems fail when medications are prescribed into a void, hoping patients will figure it out alone."***
>
> ***—Dr. Megha Poddar, Cofounder, nymble***

Wayne, Three Weeks Later

It is a Wednesday at the office. Wayne is at his desk. His phone vibrates at 11:45 (see Figure 14.2).

NYMBLE

Lunch in 15.

He keeps writing. At 12:00 it vibrates again.

NYMBLE

Grab your lunch.

He stands, walks to the office kitchen, opens the container Linda packed the night before, and sits at the small table by the window. He eats. He goes back to his desk. On the drive home that evening, he dictates a short note.

WAYNE

Ate. Five for five this week.

NYMBLE

Want to keep the 11:45 nudge, or drop it?

WAYNE

Drop it. Noon is enough.

NYMBLE

Done.

Figure 14.2 After lunch with nymble.

ENDNOTES

1. Albert Bandura, *Self-Efficacy: The Exercise of Control* (W. H. Freeman, 1997).
2. Edward L. Deci and Richard M. Ryan, *Intrinsic Motivation and Self-Determination in Human Behavior* (Plenum, 1985).
3. Judith H. Hibbard et al., "Development of the Patient Activation Measure (PAM): Conceptualizing and Measuring Activation in Patients and Consumers," *Health Services Research* 39, no. 4 Pt 1 (2004): 1005–26, https://doi.org/10.1111/j.1475-6773.2004.00269.x.
4. N. Powley et al., "Effect of Digital Health Coaching on Self-Efficacy and Lifestyle Change," *Bja Open* 4 (October 2022): 100067, https://doi.org/10.1016/j.bjao.2022.100067; Nicola Powley et al., "Digital Health Coaching to Improve Patient Preparedness for Elective Lower Limb Arthroplasty: A Quality Improvement Project," *BMJ Open Quality* 12, no. 4 (2023): e002244, https://doi.org/10.1136/bmjoq-2022-002244.
5. Aaron Severs, *Retention, Renewal, Results: Noom's GLP-1 Companion*, Noom, Noom Program, February 4, 2026, https://www.noom.com/blog/weight-management/2025-was-the-breakout-year-for-nooms-glp1-companion/.

CHAPTER 15

COMMUNITY IN THE CANOPY

Sarah is in the meat aisle on Sunday morning, looking at chicken that she does not want to cook, let alone eat. Her cart has four items. She has been in the store for 45 minutes. She has not made a decision about a single meal to prepare this week. She pulls out her phone and opens the Community app. I started it as a companion to my practice and synchronous group sessions. Sarah pauses, then asks for the help she needs (see Figure 15.1).

By the time Sarah does another loop around the aisles, six members have responded. She buys some firm tofu, rice noodles, carrots, and peanut sauce. She

Sarah

I don't know what to prepare for the week. The food I want now just doesn't seem appetizing when it gets to later in the week, and I'm really struggling not to waste food but also get excited about it. Anyone else?

Marisol

Same. I freeze portions the day I cook. Sunday-Sarah can't predict Wednesday-Sarah's appetite anymore, and that's hard to work around. What if you bought one fresh thing for now and one frozen-friendly thing for later?

Devra

I made the mistake last month of cooking a large salmon for meals. I love salmon but I could not even be around it and my husband had to finish preparing it. Thank goodness we had neighbors over so none of it went to waste. I find that cooking something I know I want on the day I want it works, but then make enough to eat the next day too.

Anita

I am so glad you posted this. I thought I was the only one. I have been throwing out so much food and feeling guilty about it on top of everything else.

Marisol

You're not the only one! Welcome.

Figure 15.1 Peers help Sarah feel seen.

thinks she wants a basic, warm Thai dish and has everything else she needs at home. The thought of chicken turned her stomach. But the tofu seemed fine. She felt better knowing that she isn't crazy and that there are others retraining their palate from scratch. She drives home to cook and share her win with the Community.

BIAS BUSTING

As a graduate student and early in my medical career, I worked alongside many people with addictions. I studied how women with addictions who were also engaged in sex work make contact with healthcare services.[1] I codesigned collaborative health research[2] and set up better access points for treatment in my local emergency room.[3] Time and again, I found that healthcare workers endorsed by other members of informal networks could more easily offer support to the whole network. In my research, I learned a great deal from members and staff at The PACE Society (a Vancouver peer-driven nonprofit that helps maintain and strengthen networks of sex workers to help them stay safe). On their website, a member describes PACE as "*somewhere I am respected, somewhere my body gets to rest*."[4]

My clinical transition to working with people with obesity may seem strange until you see how much these patient groups have in common, both socially and biologically. Bias toward people with addictions and toward people with obesity is the rule, not the exception. This remains true in 2026, even as biases around gender, sexuality, class, ethnicity, and other identities have gone underground.[5] Both diseases are very socially isolating. They close doors on jobs, relationships, travel, social rituals, and more. People with either condition hold a great deal of self-directed blame and shame despite the fact that both have a large inherited risk. Some people are more likely to develop addiction than others, all else being equal, because of their genes. The same is true for obesity, where body size is between 40% and 70% inherited.[6] Both conditions can be incited by traumatic experiences in early life, and both can emerge from experiences with the medical system itself.

To belong, a patient needs to make sense of their own experiences in relation to those of others in the network. When I ask my patients what helps them feel safe in our practice, they usually cite the *group* as a leading reason. They are referring to their weekly psychotherapy group, which is a bedrock of my practice, and our patient-only online community. When they are just starting out, patients consistently tell me they feel like they are the only ones who struggle with appetite and weight gain. I do not take on the challenge of convincing them this is not true. The group does this more elegantly and swiftly than I ever could. The longest-running groups are a safe haven from the social storm of being in a large body and all that this has come to mean. The groups are where *they* go to rest.

HELPING HELPS HELPERS, TOO

Community is not cheerleading. It is for peer identity work. Helping people with the same problem you have changes how you relate to the problem. Helping is the active ingredient of Community.

Social scientist Frank Riessman named peers as the key to addiction treatment. "People who share the same problem or condition," he wrote, "are more likely to listen to each other than to listen to professionals."[7] The line he attributes to Alcoholics Anonymous (AA) cofounder Bill Wilson is, "Drunks don't need a drink. They need a drunk." Riessman called it *helper-therapy*: the idea that the person doing the helping gains more from the involvement than the person being helped. The 2020 Cochrane review of AA-style programs showed that abstinence from alcohol was higher than in comparators.[8] Medicine has historically struggled to manage obesity and addiction, even when great medical treatments are available, because they need to be deployed inside transformation infrastructure. This includes peers in Community. Studies of sponsorship in AA find higher odds of sustained abstinence among sponsors.[9]

Peer support in digital health is different from professional support. The peer-to-peer relationship is built on mutual aid, where the helper and the helped are reciprocally engaged, and the helper benefits from the relationship in ways a clinician cannot.[10] Peer support has three parts: goal setting by the person being helped, task agreement built on shared life experiences, and a bond formed through similarity rather than professional authority. Peer support is chronic disease care, not a bell-and-whistle add-on.

MORE THAN A BULLETIN BOARD

Forming a healthy and supportive Community, especially on a digital platform, is not simple. The alchemy of Community requires an engaged, long-standing peer group, even if it is small, that knows how to welcome newcomers—because they do not always arrive ready to participate. At the start, they lurk. Lurking is when a member is in a digital Community but does not contribute. Badreddine and Blount's study of lurking in an online cancer community asked what kept lurkers silent: posts that went unanswered, moderators who were not visibly active, and peer support that did not materialize. The lurkers reported bad first experiences, a weaker sense of belonging, and lower psychological well-being than the posters (see KPI 25—time to first peer-directed act).[11]

Crossing the threshold from lurker to poster is the highest-leverage early behavior a Community can produce. Compress the median from weeks to days to demonstrate community well-being (see KPI 26—newcomer first-response time).

KPI 25 OF 50

COMPONENT	LENS	TIER
COMMUNITY	**PATIENT BEHAVIOR**	**EXPERIENCE**

KPI **TIME TO FIRST PEER-DIRECTED ACT**

Median days from a new member's enrollment to her first peer-directed act inside the community (a post, a reply, a reaction, or a direct message to another member).

MEASURES	Whether the community's onboarding, tone, and visible activity converted a new member from lurker to participant, and how quickly.
SIGNAL	Short medians indicate Community maturity and thoughtful workflows. Long medians (multi-week, multi-month) indicate intimidation, inactivity, or irrelevance.
TIMEFRAME	First 30 days after enrollment.

KPI 26 OF 50

COMPONENT	LENS	TIER
COMMUNITY	**PROGRAM STEWARDSHIP**	**EXPERIENCE**

KPI **NEWCOMER FIRST-RESPONSE TIME**

Median hours from a newcomer's first post to first substantive response (from a peer, moderator, help-giver, or clinical team member).

MEASURES	Whether the program has staffed, tooled, and culturally primed the community to answer new voices.
SIGNAL	Short medians and low 72-hour no-response rates indicate active stewardship.
TIMEFRAME	Per newcomer post, first ninety days of membership.

What counts as a substantive response was established in Chapter 14 by the substantive response rule to include informational content, emotional support, specific acknowledgment, or advocacy. The response has to feel, and actually be, real.

THE PEER OWNERSHIP PIVOT

After the first month, newcomers should organically shift into a peer identity (see KPI 27—help-giver activation rate).

Helper rate is the observable, countable signature of emerging peer identity. A patient who answers another patient's first post at 8:00 in the morning—before their own coffee, on their own time, with their own hard-won knowledge—is showing up for their Community in a way that helps everyone. The program design imperative is to normalize high-quality member contribution, alongside healthy professional moderation, to deepen engagement (see KPI 28—member content rate).

KPI 27 OF 50

COMPONENT	LENS	TIER
COMMUNITY	**PATIENT BEHAVIOR**	**ENGAGEMENT**

KPI **HELP-GIVER ACTIVATION RATE**

Percentage of active patients with at least one help-giving act per month.

MEASURES	Whether the community is producing the identity pivot that the helper-therapy literature predicts is durable.
SIGNAL	Rising rates indicate identity work at scale.
TIMEFRAME	Measured monthly; trended across months two through twelve. One count per patient per month.

KPI 28 OF 50

COMPONENT	LENS	TIER
COMMUNITY	**PROGRAM STEWARDSHIP**	**ENGAGEMENT**

KPI **MEMBER CONTENT RATE**

Percentage of total content created by members (not moderators).

MEASURES	**How much of the Community conversation is driven by members versus the program team.**
SIGNAL	**A rising Member : Moderator content ratio means feeling safe in and ownership of the Community.**
TIMEFRAME	**Tracked monthly, reported as a monthly rate by cohort.**

LIVY'S PELOTON

Peloton leaned on its Community to come back from the brink I described in Chapter 6.[12] Their Community infrastructure has live synchronous and asynchronous elements that mutually reinforce its health. During live classes, riders high-five each other while the instructor coaches, DJs, and narrates the leaderboard out loud to stoke competition. Outside of workouts, there is a peer-driven menu of ways to be in Community, including real-life cycling clubs, popular Reddit threads and Facebook groups, post-class messages, and milestone celebrations in the Peloton app.[13]

The Livy Method is a Canadian-built health and wellness program that comprises 360,000 cumulative members across more than 55 countries.[14] Founder Gina Livy ran fitness studios and was a weight-loss coach for decades before pivoting to an online Community model in 2018. The Livy Method's asynchronous and synchronous elements create constant opportunities for members to interact with one another and Livy moderators, including Gina Livy herself.[15] Members join cohorts, so they share milestones and a daily cadence of well-timed content to reinforce habits. Members disclose difficulties to their cohorts because of a built-in anti-shame framework that guides moderation. Dr. Ruth Kane at the University of Ottawa frames the Livy Method explicitly as a community of practice, a term from education theory describing learning that happens through social participation among people with shared goals.[16] Members on their second or third cycle sit beside first-time members, which organically fosters peer helping.

Gina Livy is the gravitational center of the Livy Method. She does daily livestreams to the members. Her own weight-loss origin story positions her immediately as a trusted peer. Similarly, Peloton's instructors are minor celebrities with whom riders describe a one-sided bond that feels like friendship. That bond is what makes synchronous elements so powerful, but it is also a source of program fragility. Communities should build the synchronous layer around teams of experts and the asynchronous layer around peers who become helpers. This flywheel of helpers reinforces the fabric of Community for the next cohort of newcomers.

SARAH IN THE COMMUNITY

Sarah noticed how good it felt to share her struggle and have her experience validated by the Community. She was initially hesitant; interested enough to lurk but not yet confident enough to contribute. Day after day, she kept opening the Community to see what people shared. She found it more supportive and useful than expected. Eventually, she signed up for a live question-and-answer session with her cohort's dietitian to get more meal inspiration.

ENDNOTES

1. Ashley White, "Making Outreach Matter: Investigating Health Service Assets for Sex Workers Who Inject Drugs in Vancouver's Downtown Eastside," International Harm Reduction Conference, Bangkok, 2009.
2. Lisa Lazarus et al., "Community Engagement and Ownership in the Development and Design of PROUD, an Ottawa CBPR Study," Canadian Association for HIV/AIDS Research 2013, Vancouver, May 2013; Yoko S. Schreiber et al., "Using Respondent-Driven Sampling to Access People Who Use Drugs in Ottawa-Gatineau: Practical and Ethical Considerations," Canadian Association for HIV/AIDS Research 2013, Vancouver, May 2013.
3. Ellen Buck-McFadyen et al., "Pilot Program Integrating Outpatient Opioid Treatment within a Rural Primary Care Setting," *Rural and Remote Health* 21, no. 3 (2021), https://doi.org/10.22605/RRH6413.
4. Anonymous, PACE member, "PACE Society—By, With & For Sex Workers Since 1994," PACE, accessed May 14, 2026, https://www.pace-society.org/.
5. Sean Wharton et al., "Obesity in Adults: A Clinical Practice Guideline," Guideline, *Canadian Medical Association Journal* 192, no. 31 (2020): E875–91, https://doi.org/10.1503/cmaj.191707.
6. Ruth J. F. Loos and Giles S. H. Yeo, "The Genetics of Obesity: From Discovery to Biology," *Nature Reviews Genetics* 23, no. 2 (2022): 120–33, https://doi.org/10.1038/s41576-021-00414-z.
7. Frank Riessman, "The Peer Principle: The Key to Addiction Treatment," *Social Policy* 29, no. 2 (1998): 10–13.
8. John F. Kelly et al., *Alcoholics Anonymous and Other 12-Step Programs for Alcohol Use Disorder—Kelly, JF—2020 | Cochrane Library*, n.d., accessed May 14, 2026, https://www.cochranelibrary.com/cdsr/doi/10.1002/14651858.CD012880.pub2/full.
9. Byron L. Crape et al., "The Effects of Sponsorship in 12-Step Treatment of Injection Drug Users," *Drug and Alcohol Dependence* 65, no. 3 (2002): 291–301, https://doi.org/10.1016/s0376-8716(01)00175-2.
10. Karen L. Fortuna et al., "Peer Support: A Human Factor to Enhance Engagement in Digital Health Behavior Change Interventions," *Journal of Technology in Behavioral Science* 4, no. 2 (2019): 152–61, https://doi.org/10.1007/s41347-019-00105-x.
11. Basma M. Badreddine and Yvette Blount, "Understanding Influential Factors Behind Lurking Behaviour in Online Cancer Communities," *Behaviour & Information Technology* 40, no. 6 (2021): 542–64, https://doi.org/10.1080/0144929X.2019.1709545.
12. Shashank Srinivasan et al., *Peloton Interactive (A)*, no. 9-323-005 (Boston: Harvard Business School Publishing, 2025); Joshua Foster and Ryan Cheng, *Peloton Interactive Inc.: A Push to Keep Users Pedalling*, no. W35254 (Ivey Publishing, Ivey Business School, Western University, 2024).

13. "These Peloton Community Features Will Help You Stay Connected," Peloton, *The Output*, July 22, 2025, https://www.onepeloton.com/blog/peloton-community-features; Liz Doupnik, "How to Make the Most of Your Online Fitness Community," Peloton, *The Output*, May 1, 2025, https://www.onepeloton.com/blog/online-fitness-community.
14. "Meet Gina Livy," The Livy Method, accessed May 14, 2026, https://livymethod.com/pages/meet-gina-livy; CanadianSME, *Gina Livy on Redefining Sustainable Weight Loss*, CanadianSME Business Magazine, December 16, 2025, https://canadiansme.ca/gina-livy-on-redefining-sustainable-weight-loss/.
15. "The Livy Method," The Livy Method, accessed May 14, 2026, https://livymethod.com/.
16. Gina Livy and Ruth Kane, *Researching The Livy Method as a Community of Practice* (Gina Livy, 2024), YouTube video, 14:48, https://www.youtube.com/watch?v=u7CvEpO5GOo.

CHAPTER 16

CONNECTION IN THE CANOPY

Some of the images in this chapter are too large or complex to properly format in printed form. Figures marked with a WAV label can be downloaded from the Web Added Value Download Resource Center at www.jrosspub.com/wav for proper viewing.

"I'm happy with where I am weight-wise," Sarah shares, "and I'd like to talk about the plan from here."

Sarah walks me through her numbers. Based on her age, weight, sex, and activity level, she knows how much she needs to eat each day to maintain her weight. This is her total daily energy expenditure (TDEE). It is the same number Wayne calculated in Chapter 13. Based on her twice-weekly food logs, her daily intake is within this range while taking 1 mg of semaglutide per week. "I don't want to be frail at sixty," she says. "I want to be strong." This is a different Sarah from the one who walked into my office two years ago with a giant bag of supplements and a spreadsheet of macros. That Sarah was looking for a code to crack. This one knows what she wants and how to pace herself (see Figure 16.1).

When she looks at it all laid out like this, it feels very doable. I updated her Care plan and renewed her prescriptions for semaglutide, estradiol patch, and progesterone. We plan her next visit for two months from now. The systems my practice uses keep Sarah, my team, and me connected between visits, in case we need to make an adjustment. It's here, in *Connection*, where we can imagine the dovetailing of patient and health system transformation.

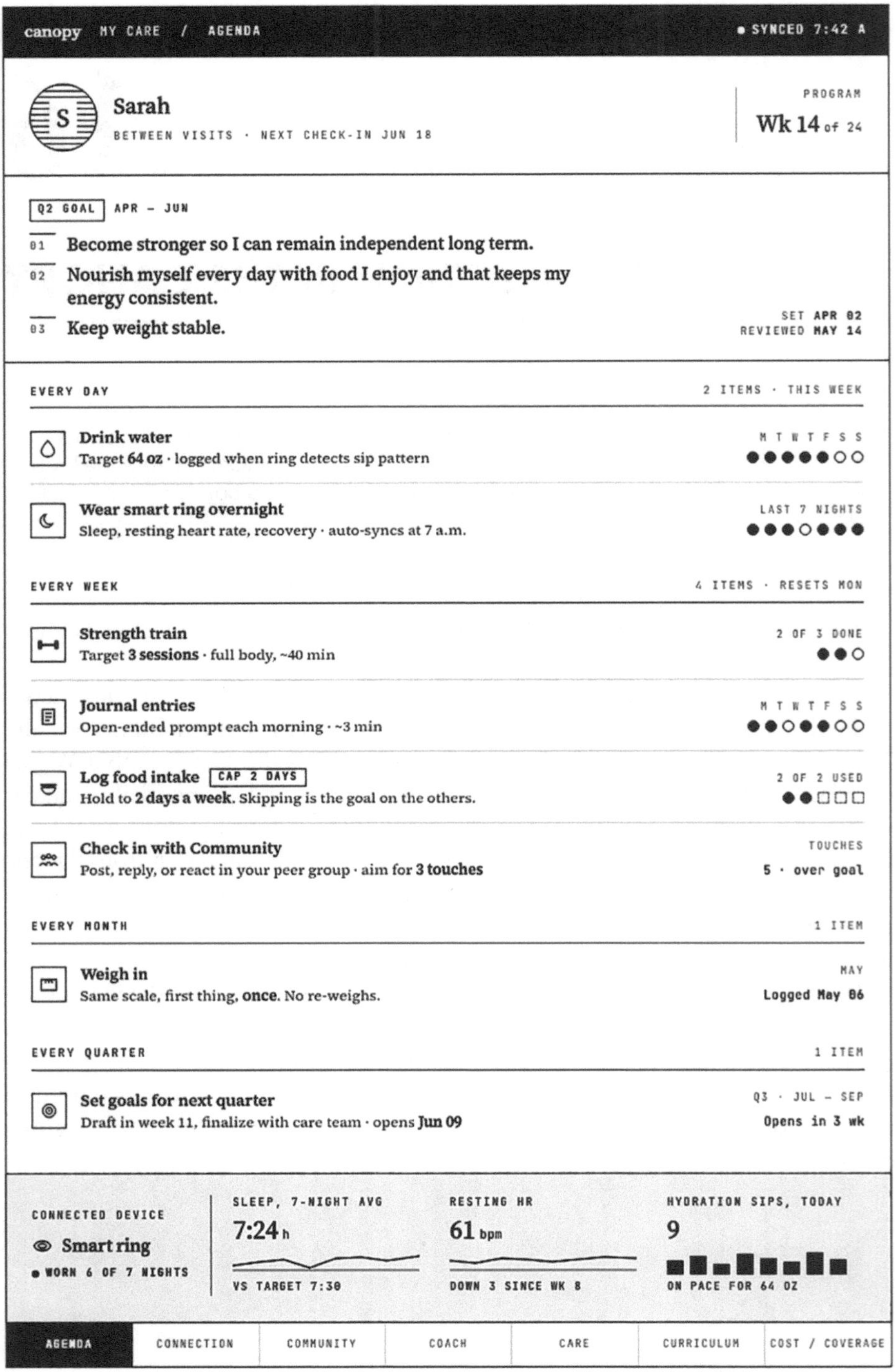

Figure 16.1 Sarah's patient agenda.

LISTENING BETWEEN VISITS

What follows shows how Connection in the Canopy could look when handling a common stress test in obesity medicine. A month after Sarah leaves my office, I get a notification (see Figure 16.2).

I read this synthesis in under a minute and know exactly what's going on. In a typical practice, the drag on our time is in gathering and organizing the data for the way we actually think, and to protect our minds from systematic biases. Once you're experienced enough, decisions come quickly.

It would have taken me 20 minutes to reconstruct this straight from her chart on my own. It would have taken a senior resident about an hour to gather everything relevant to present this case to me from across multiple clunky digital portals. Instead, the Canopy can pull everything relevant and assemble it for clinician review.

The chart shows her gallbladder still in place and potential contributions from her medication list. Her journals from the last three weeks mention reflux and bloating, which she has not yet flagged to Care. Since chicken wing night, Sarah has been avoiding dinner to see if she can manage on her own, but she's undereating. She may think this is temporary, but to my expert eyes, it's only going to stop when her gallbladder comes out.

Empowered patients are a double-edged sword. They are keen to piece together their experience and understand what is happening. Sarah trusts me to take her seriously. I always have. She knows that when she wants my help, she will get it. Connection is helping her, and I come back to Care to help build a better shared awareness. I can't initiate this on my own for thousands of patients. And Sarah won't bring every little sensation to me in a visit, nor should she, but she should write it down so that patterns can be seen. Connection solves for the reality and human psychology of it all.

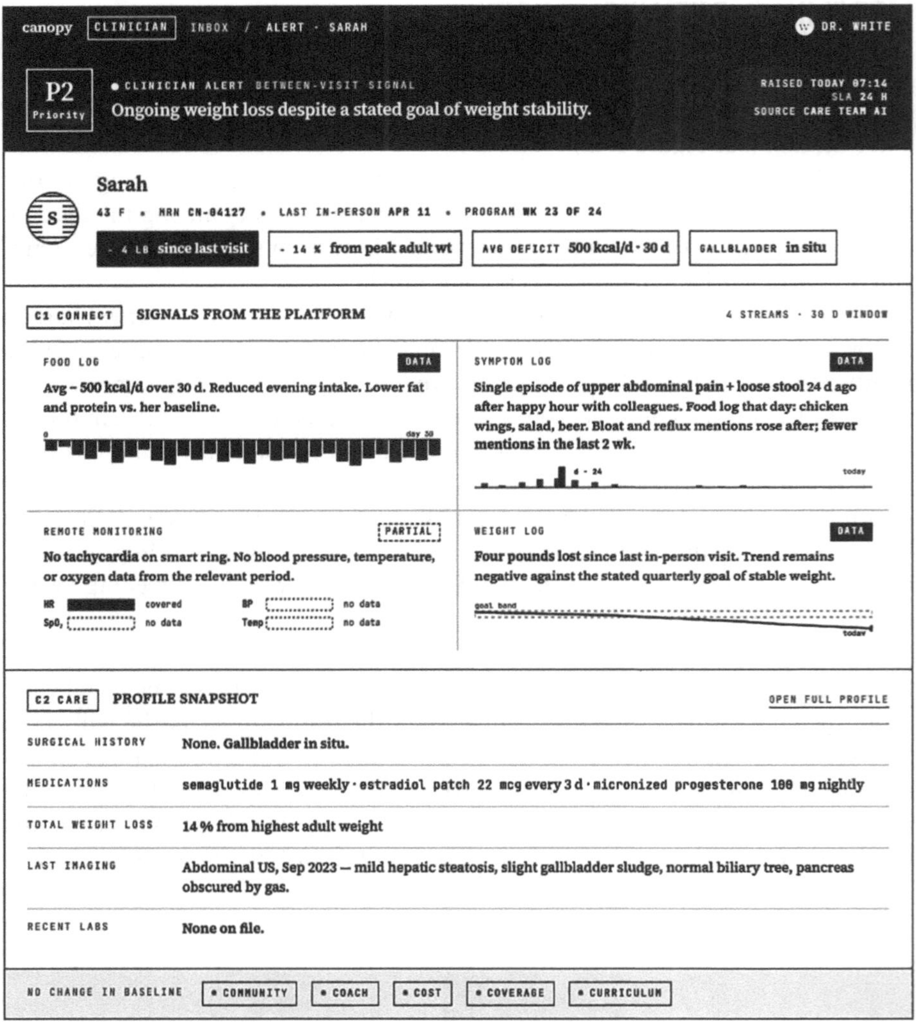

Figure 16.2 Clinician alert for Sarah. *(art continued on next page.)*

WHAT WOULD THE MONOCROP DO?

Here is how this exact scenario plays out *without* Connection in the Canopy. Sarah loses more weight than intended because she is avoiding fullness, spices, and fatty foods. At her monthly refill, she receives a congratulatory message about her weight loss because they do not know her agenda includes weight stability. They don't ask

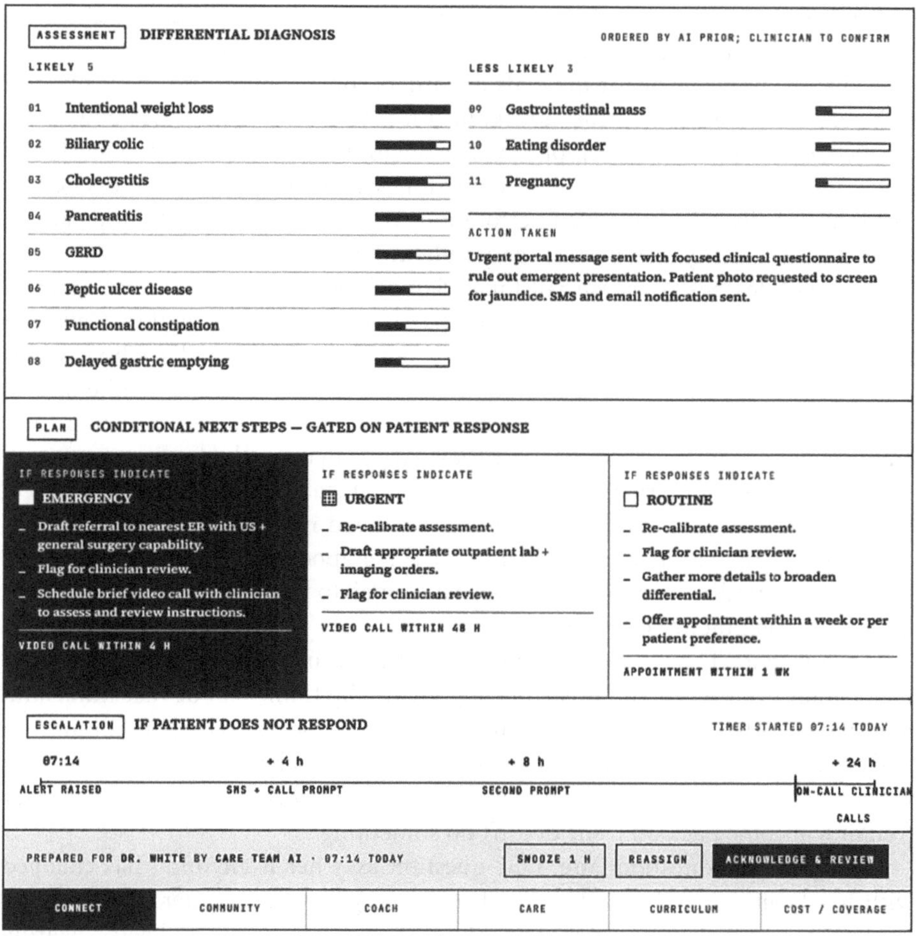

Figure 16.2 *continued*

if she's having side effects. So, she doesn't tell them because she is handling it. Her prescription is auto-titrated to 1.7 mg of semaglutide, and they don't know about her hormone therapy.

A few weeks later, she experiences sudden, incapacitating pain in her upper abdomen. She's terrified. She messages her platform but gets nowhere. She calls 911 and is taken to the emergency department. The triage nurse asks her to recite all of her medications and doses before she gets any pain relief. "Semaglutide 1.7 mg per week," she mutters before the nurse, shaking her head, interrupts her, "Oh, that stuff. Terrible!"

Sarah is overcome with shame and wants to disappear into her stretcher. *She thinks I did this to myself*; she frets, *they're going to think I'm faking it.*

A doctor evaluates her at the bedside, orders some testing, and she waits. She isn't sure if she's having a heart attack, or if it is pancreatitis, or if her bowels are blocked, or something else completely. The doctor returns with results a few hours later: "It's your gallbladder. You have some stones, and it looks like it has opened up inside your belly, which is called perforation. We see this with semaglutide all the time; it is really risky. You need surgery right away."

Semaglutide does not cause gallstones. Semaglutide causes weight loss, and significant weight loss by any means is a risk factor for gallstone formation. Gallstone formation is a risk factor for cholecystitis, or an inflamed gallbladder. Cholecystitis is a risk factor for gallbladder perforation. But this chain of events is neither causal nor inevitable. My colleagues in the emergency department can over-anchor their biases in worst-case scenarios because they have to manage them.

Sarah has her surgery and recovers at home. It takes her a few weeks to feel normal, but by week three, her appetite is back and insatiable. She figures it has something to do with her gallbladder because her appetite wasn't even this strong before she started semaglutide. She opens her email to find an auto-reminder from her monocrop practice (see Figure 16.3).

Sarah is livid. They didn't help her when she was in crisis. They increased her medication even when she wasn't feeling great. She thinks about that nurse and how bad it felt to know that they might have thought she was taking up room from *real emergencies* for something she did to herself. She wishes she could manage her weight without medication, but her appetite is so strong right now. She knows her weight will come back on if she doesn't do something.

She opens the questionnaire. One question asks her if anything has changed with her health since her last refill. "I had emergency gallbladder surgery three weeks ago, and they removed it." She submits her questionnaire and gets a weirdly rapid response:

"We're sorry—you have indicated that you have a medical condition that makes you ineligible for further treatment with us. Please follow up with your general practitioner."

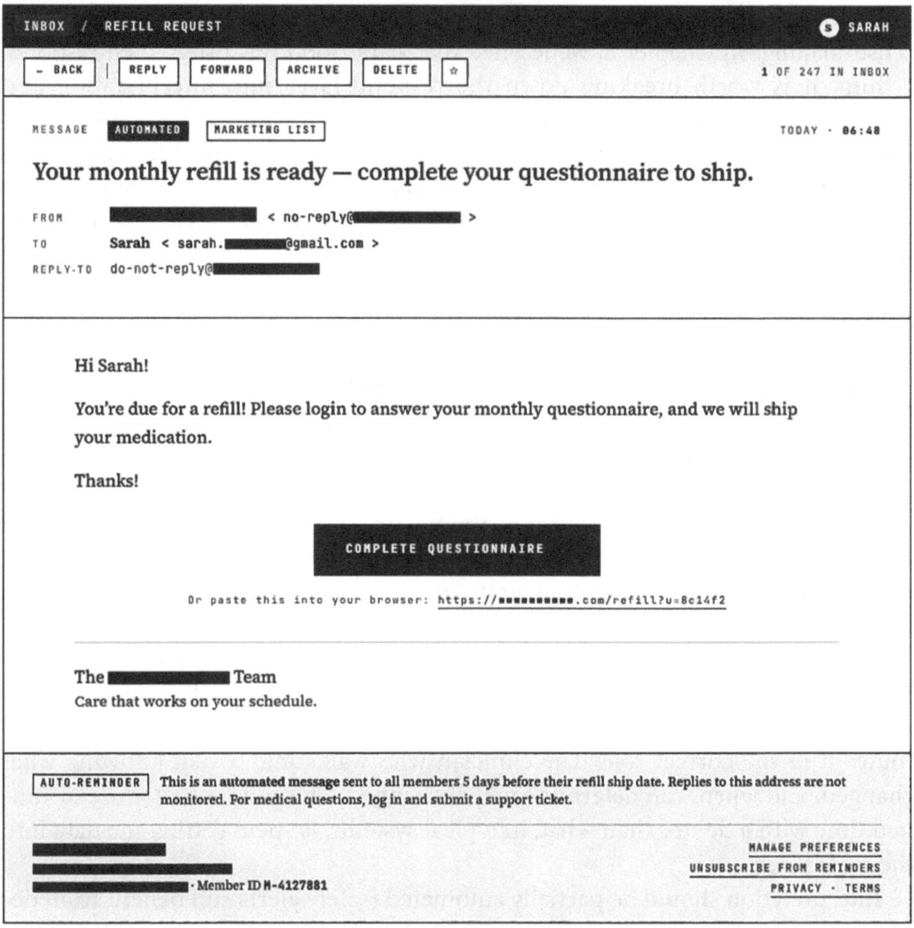

INBOX / REFILL REQUEST

S SARAH

← BACK | REPLY | FORWARD | ARCHIVE | DELETE | ☆

1 OF 247 IN INBOX

MESSAGE AUTOMATED MARKETING LIST

TODAY · 06:48

Your monthly refill is ready — complete your questionnaire to ship.

FROM [redacted] < no-reply@[redacted] >

TO Sarah < sarah.[redacted]@gmail.com >

REPLY-TO do-not-reply@[redacted]

Hi Sarah!

You're due for a refill! Please login to answer your monthly questionnaire, and we will ship your medication.

Thanks!

COMPLETE QUESTIONNAIRE

Or paste this into your browser: https://[redacted].com/refill?u=8c14f2

The [redacted] Team

Care that works on your schedule.

AUTO-REMINDER This is an automated message sent to all members 5 days before their refill ship date. Replies to this address are not monitored. For medical questions, log in and submit a support ticket.

[redacted] · Member ID M-4127881

MANAGE PREFERENCES

UNSUBSCRIBE FROM REMINDERS

PRIVACY · TERMS

Figure 16.3 Standard refill request outside of the Canopy.

LISTENING, INTERPRETATION, AND SENSE-MAKING

The traditional medical model is not much better and cannot accommodate the scale of systemic obesity care we need. Chronic diseases, like obesity, progress between doctor visits. In Novo Nordisk's 2026 *State of Weight and Health Report*, 94% of healthcare providers said they actively listen to patients with obesity without judgment. Only 39% of people with obesity agreed.[1] Closing this 55-point gap does not come from trying harder inside existing systems. It comes from building Connection.

There are three parts of a Connection loop: listening, interpretation, and sense-making. In Chapter 8, we learned that Zara's loop was listen, then respond. I think it is worth breaking down the respond layer into interpretation and sense-making. Because the Canopy integrates patient learning (Curriculum), peer interaction (Community), medication (Care), and growth (Coach), the Connection component can pass a signal through multiple components. This makes the signal meaningful to the system (interpretation) and to who really matters here: the patient.

Listening is structured signal capture between visits. Which signals matter? This depends on the patient, but WAV Figure 16.4 is a non-exhaustive list of what I listen to, depending on the patient and their consent. Together, there are thousands of potential variables and millions of data points for each. No system should begin with all of this. The KPIs for Connection incentivize programs to select a few narrow listening channels, design well around them, and then add more channels.

This data flows back into the patient's own Care, and the patient chooses what to connect and at what cadence. That distinction is what separates a listening system from a surveillance system. A listening system gathers all of this, along with the patient's own annotations, and integrates it for the benefit of both the patient and the clinician.

Interpretation turns a raw signal into clinical meaning. A declining food-log frequency could indicate appetite dysregulation, travel events, schedule chaos, loss of motivation, or hospitalization. The interpretation layer reveals what matters and routes it to the correct role. The clinician who walks into a visit knowing what changed, and when, can determine why it changed. This is a far better use of limited time with a doctor than what, in typical systems, is spent getting the data into the right place.

Interpretation should be partially automated (safety alerts still benefit from deterministic branching logic while the slower thinking systems formulate below the surface), semi-autonomous and intelligent (synthesizing many clinical variables from disparate parts of the record at once), and rely on human-in-the-loop so the clinician is always participating in interpretation for patients, steering based on the full humanized context.

Sense-making turns interpretation into a therapeutic intervention. Interpretation needs to be shared in a way that meets the patient where they are, ideally using stories. It has to acknowledge shame, fear, budgets, and much more. Patients on

GLP-1 therapy experience changes that unfold over months because The MAP™ (metabolism, appetite, perspective) shifts quickly and constantly. *Without* help, patients narrate them as disconnected, often frightening events. *With* help, the patient places the experience inside an arc: this is what your normal feels like, this is what appetite return means, this is what emotions look like without food to cover them up. None of it means failure. Sense-making, paired with Curriculum, helps patients learn what they need to make decisions about their lives.

CONNECTION KPIS

In the first 30 days, keep Connection simple and aim to connect the patient to just one channel at a time (see KPI 29—first signal time (FST)).

The Connection infrastructure score (see KPI 30) measures whether the design supports the listening, interpretation, and sense-making loop. The score is based on bundles of evidence-based practices that, when implemented together, support better outcomes than any single practice. Bundles come from research in critical care that shows clinicians may think they are doing all the right things, but usually are not, until each thing is measured and tracked.[2] All-or-none scoring means a bundle is counted as complete only when all elements are delivered.[3]

A closed-loop rate (see KPI 31) measures the patient's substantive engagement with interpretation. When the system surfaces a signal, routes it through interpretation, and generates outreach to the patient, the patient needs to engage within their capacity to ensure sense-making and to close the loop.

Paired with the closed-loop rate, the loop-ready outreach rate (see KPI 32) is also a bundle of elements and serves as an integrity check on the system's design. If the listening works and the interpretation is correct, but the patient has no idea what is happening, then the listening and interpretation do not matter. The outreach between interpretation and sense-making needs to set the patient up for sense-making by being *loop-ready*. Loop-ready means that communication with the patient comes from the right part of the system role or component, references the signal heard, clarifies the next steps, asks the patient to respond within a certain time window, and includes an escalation plan. The less critical the signal, the more open-ended the outreach can be.

KPI 29 OF 50

COMPONENT	LENS	TIER
CONNECTION	**PATIENT BEHAVIOR**	**EXPERIENCE**

KPI **FIRST SIGNAL TIME (FST)**

The median number of days from enrollment to the first substantive patient-initiated signal received and logged by the program. Channel-agnostic. The metric is whether listening was established.

MEASURES	Whether the patient added any form of continuous data to the system, including remote vitals, food logging, journaling, symptom reporting, scoring, or messaging.
SIGNAL	Short FST means the channels exist, are trusted, and are being used. Long FST means either the channels are missing, untrusted, or the program's response history has taught patients not to bother.
TIMEFRAME	First 30 days after enrollment.

KPI 30 OF 50

COMPONENT	LENS	TIER
CONNECTION	**PROGRAM STEWARDSHIP**	**EXPERIENCE**

KPI **CONNECTION INFRASTRUCTURE SCORE**

A binary score, 0 or 1, indicating whether the program meets all five conditions of functional Connection infrastructure. Uses all-or-none scoring; partial compliance scores zero.

CONDITIONS

(1) At least three distinct signal-capture channels, of which at least two are universal rather than tied to a specific device, app, or subscription state.

(2) A published signal taxonomy describing what the program can listen for and how each signal class is classified.

(3) A mechanism for patients to choose signals to connect and the cadence of that connection.

(4) Documented routing logic specifying which role receives each class of signals and escalation thresholds.

(5) Clinical-layer data governance for captured signals, written to the identified patient record at the time of capture.

MEASURES	Whether the design supports the listening, interpretation, and sense-making loop.
SIGNAL	Listen loops established.
TIMEFRAME	Audited annually; attested quarterly by the clinical director.

KPI 31 OF 50

COMPONENT	LENS	TIER
CONNECTION	**PATIENT BEHAVIOR**	**ENGAGEMENT**

KPI **CLOSED LOOP RATE**

The percentage of program-initiated outreach events where the patient engages substantively within 72 hours.

MEASURES	Whether the interpretation is becoming sense-making through substantive patient engagement.
SIGNAL	Mature programs see CLR rise across cohorts as the loops of Connection deepen.
TIMEFRAME	Rolling 30-day window. Reported monthly.

KPI 32 OF 50

COMPONENT	LENS	TIER
CONNECTION	**PROGRAM STEWARDSHIP**	**ENGAGEMENT**

KPI **LOOP-READY OUTREACH RATE (LOR)**

The percentage of outreach events meeting all five elements of loop-ready outreach (signal-referenced, action-clear, response-windowed, role-matched, escalation plan), scored all-or-none.

ELEMENTS

(1) Signal-referenced — the outreach names the specific signal that prompted it.

(2) Action-clear — the patient can complete specific actions inside the message.

(3) Response-windowed — the outreach names when a response is expected.

(4) Role-matched — the sending role or system component is named and is appropriate for the signal class and urgency.

(5) Escalation-ready — if there is no response from the patient, the sender has a tiered plan to escalate as needed.

MEASURES	Whether outreach between interpretation and sense-making sets the patient up to close the loop.
SIGNAL	Mature programs scale listening only after being confident in the loop-readiness of existing channels.
TIMEFRAME	Audited monthly; sampled quarterly with stratification across outreach types.

BIG LEARNING COMES FROM BIG LISTENING

The listening, interpretation, and sense-making loop also occurs at the aggregate level. Drug development requires a strict sequence:

1. Basic research
2. Preclinical testing
3. Phase I clinical trials
4. Phase II clinical trials
5. Phase III clinical trials
6. Regulatory review
7. Commercial launch

This process evolved for good reasons. Safety demands extensive testing before a medication reaches large numbers of people. Both researchers and regulators require controlled conditions. The alternative would be worse. Releasing medications without this rigor creates more harm than release delays, outside of rare public health emergencies.

Both Eli Lilly and Novo Nordisk have invested heavily in AI and machine learning to speed drug discovery, compressing timelines that once stretched decades. But faster discovery does not solve for that *second moment of truth* mentioned in Chapter 4. What happens after a medication is available for use? What can we learn, and how, from real-world use?

I see this gap in my own practice. The clinical trials predicted nausea and gastrointestinal symptoms to watch for. They did not track the bureaucratic exhaustion from fighting prior-authorization denials. They did not capture the cognitive load of navigating coverage gaps. They did not prepare clinicians for the constant viral GLP-1 disinformation our patients contemplate every day on social media. The trials measured what they were designed to measure. Patients leave for reasons the system was never built to hear.

Both Novo Nordisk and Eli Lilly have made sincere attempts to understand patient experience beyond clinical trial endpoints. Evidation is a health-data company that recruits large cohorts of consenting participants, collects behavioral and physiological signals from their smartphones and wearables, and sells the resulting analyses to pharmaceutical partners. The company reports five million individual participants across the United States.[4] Its largest partnership is with Eli Lilly, a collaboration that expanded in 2018 to include obesity and GLP-1 research.[5]

In December 2025, Evidation published findings from a survey of more than 60,000 of its participants actively managing their weight.[6] One in seven of those taking injectable GLP-1s were *microdosing*: deliberately splitting or reducing their prescribed dose to manage tolerability, reduce costs, and transition to weight maintenance. Nearly a third of those not on GLP-1 medications expressed interest in microdosing motivated by cost, concerns about muscle loss, and a desire for greater dose flexibility. They also shared that, for the most part, they are getting information about microdosing from social media rather than discussing it with their clinicians. Some patients are afraid of their clinician's judgment, which is a valid concern. Others can't reach their clinician to have these discussions, which is also valid. Connection helps us bridge the enormous chasms between the clinical ideal and the patient's reality.

Every patient signal is a sacred form of personal health information. It belongs to the patient, is written to the patient's record at the time of capture, and is governed under each jurisdiction's rules for personal and health data.[7] When patients register for a health program, they need to understand and agree to how their data will be used. In a monocrop platform, microdosing breaks refill workflows and compromises branded medication margins. Therefore, they don't talk about it or design for it outside of compounding. Evidation obtained patient consent to examine the gap between how the medications are prescribed and how they are used. When microdosing is invisible to clinicians, we cannot counsel patients on the risks or understand their reasoning. We cannot adjust treatment plans before the practice does because it silently undermines outcomes and creates complications.

The ways in which we use, collect, segment, and learn from health data are about to undergo a dramatic change. They are tethered to the past only by laws unlikely to keep pace with the industry's use of AI. Personal health data must, under U.S. law, clear one of three pathways before it can be used for reasons other than the individual's care. They are highly simplified here:

1. De-identify the data by stripping 18 specific identifiers (such as name, month and day of birth, etc.)
2. Present a written authorization for the specific research purpose that has been signed by the patient
3. The use may fall under an institutional review board protocol that meets informed consent requirements

Once data have cleared one of these pathways, they can be aggregated, analyzed, and shared with research partners under a Data Use Agreement, but they can never be reidentified or connected back to the individual. Large data sets are crucial for scientific advancement: they reveal population-scale patterns that randomized trials are not designed to capture, and in real time. But that same information, unprotected, becomes a tool for steering treatment choices based on who funded the analysis for advertising, for surveillance, or for commercial interests.

The value of aggregate Connection data gives rise to a corresponding obligation; the platforms that collect it are bound to patient benefit via sense-making.

SARAH, CONNECTED

While I was reading the notification about Sarah's ongoing weight loss, Sarah received her own message (see Figure 16.5).

The message goes on to screen her for fever, jaundice, recurring pain or vomiting, and, finally, menstrual period. Sarah replies two hours later (see Figure 16.6).

The system, listening for a response, recalibrates the assessment to favor a non-emergent presentation. It prepares a draft order for blood work, urine pregnancy testing, and an ultrasound of her abdomen. Sarah gets another message (see Figure 16.7).

The symptoms do not warrant same-day imaging; the acute flags are negative. The next step is a conversation, either with me or an AI-powered diagnostic conversation tool (see Figure 16.8).

I review the case summary, then approve the draft blood testing orders and the Care plan update. I dictate a brief note to Sarah (see Figure 16.9).

The message names what we are looking for and why, in plain language, without catastrophizing. I see Sarah on Friday and find that her right upper abdomen seems to be tender when I examine her. Her blood work looks normal, and she is not pregnant. I ordered an ultrasound to be done within a few days. My system alerts me to the results (see Figure 16.10).

I check the referral draft and approve it. The system sends it and builds in automatic checks to ensure Sarah is seen in a timely manner. She is on the border between semi-urgent and urgent. Then Sarah gets the interpretation and sense-making response (see Figure 16.11).

Sarah responds right away, closing this loop (see Figure 16.12).

This is Connection. With it, we do not need to accept the trade-off between speed, affordability, clinical acumen, and humanity. Just as Zara does not confine its listening loops to one woman with a sweater in one store at one time, we should no longer settle for the rigid container of a doctor's appointment or a deterministic online questionnaire and call it healthcare.

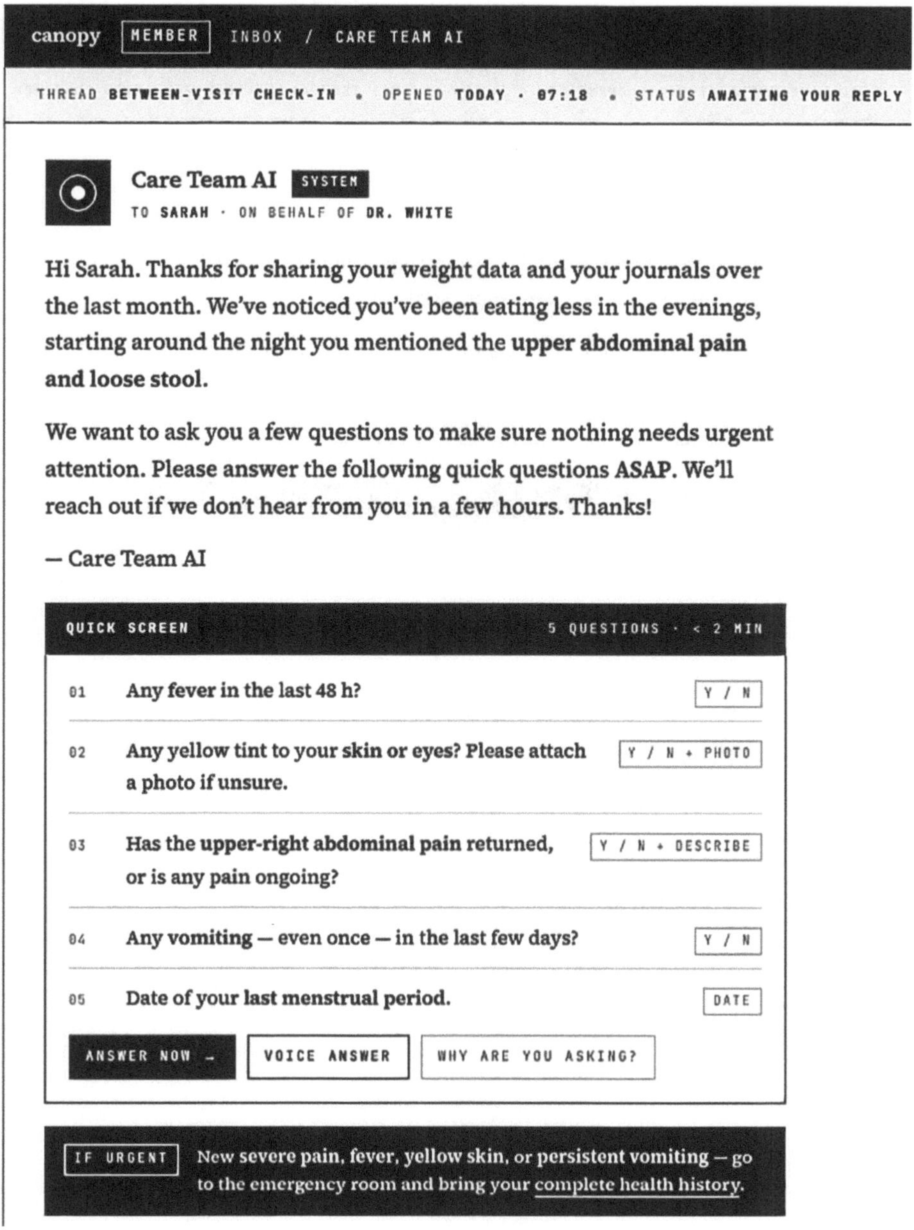

Figure 16.5 Care Team AI checks in.

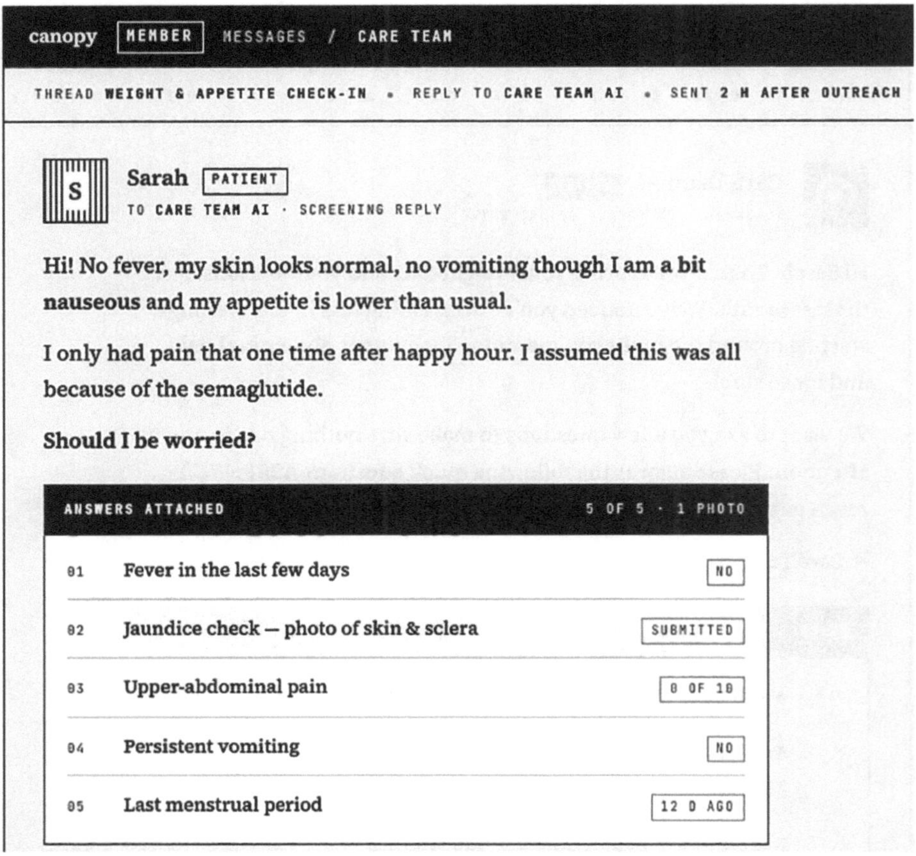

Figure 16.6 Sarah replies.

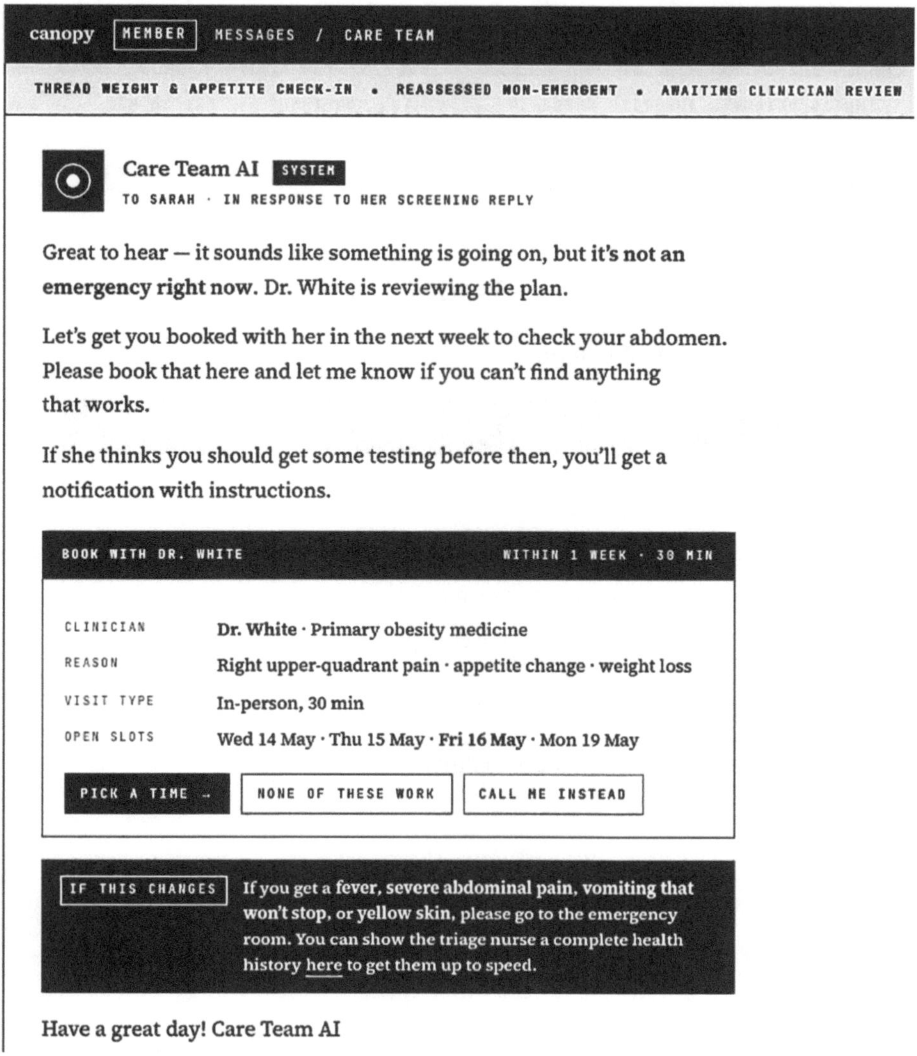

Figure 16.7 Care Team AI responds with a plan.

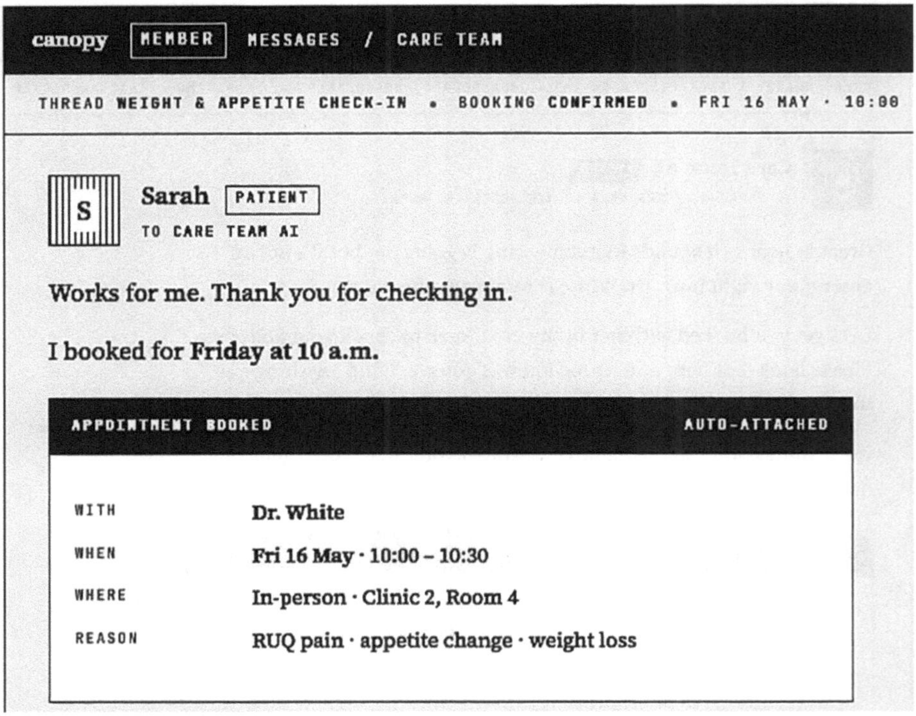

Figure 16.8 Sarah confirms her appointment.

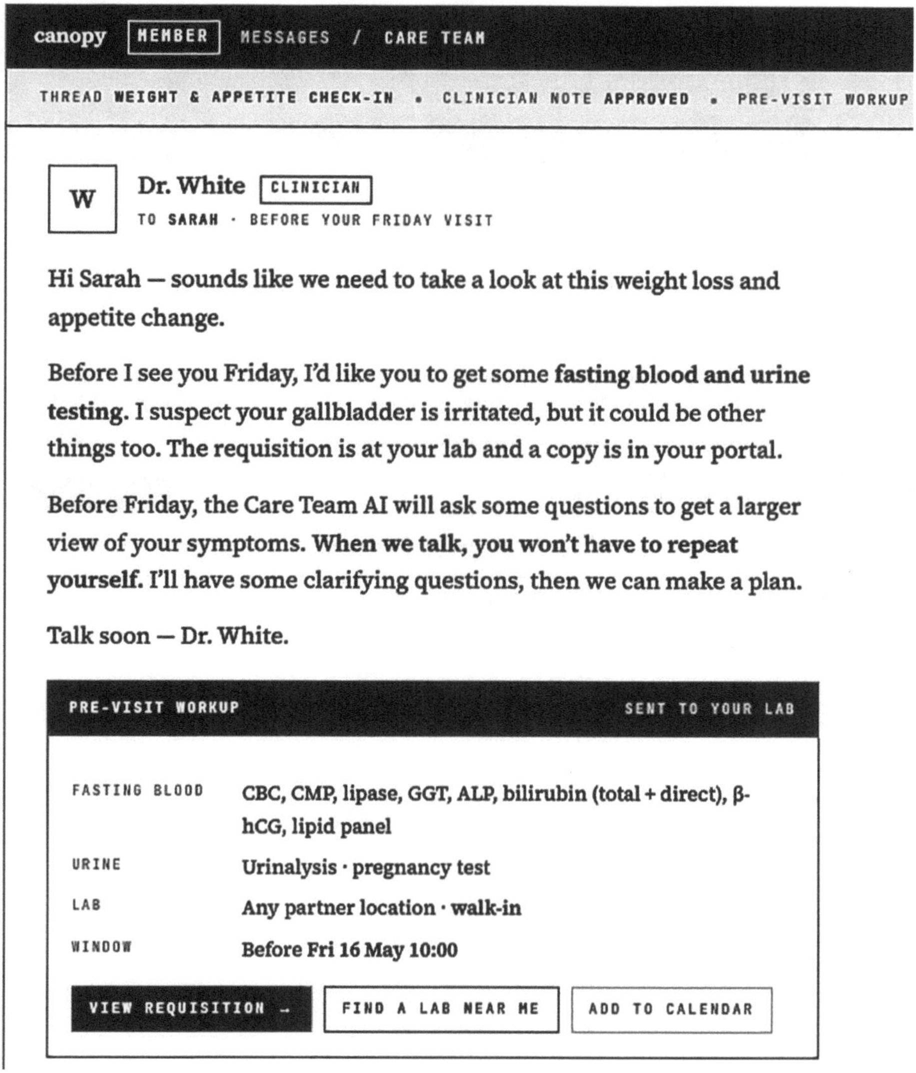

canopy MEMBER MESSAGES / CARE TEAM

THREAD WEIGHT & APPETITE CHECK-IN • CLINICIAN NOTE APPROVED • PRE-VISIT WORKUP

W

Dr. White CLINICIAN

TO SARAH · BEFORE YOUR FRIDAY VISIT

Hi Sarah — sounds like we need to take a look at this weight loss and appetite change.

Before I see you Friday, I'd like you to get some **fasting blood and urine testing.** I suspect your gallbladder is irritated, but it could be other things too. The requisition is at your lab and a copy is in your portal.

Before Friday, the Care Team AI will ask some questions to get a larger view of your symptoms. **When we talk, you won't have to repeat yourself.** I'll have some clarifying questions, then we can make a plan.

Talk soon — Dr. White.

PRE-VISIT WORKUP SENT TO YOUR LAB

FASTING BLOOD	CBC, CMP, lipase, GGT, ALP, bilirubin (total + direct), β-hCG, lipid panel
URINE	Urinalysis · pregnancy test
LAB	Any partner location · walk-in
WINDOW	Before Fri 16 May 10:00

VIEW REQUISITION → FIND A LAB NEAR ME ADD TO CALENDAR

Figure 16.9 Dr. White's note to Sarah.

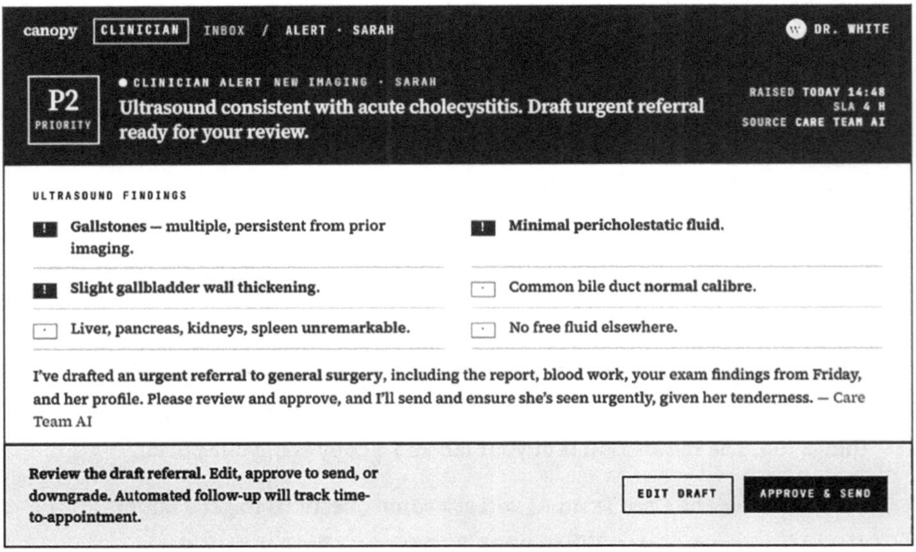

Figure 16.10 Clinician alert: Ultrasound results.

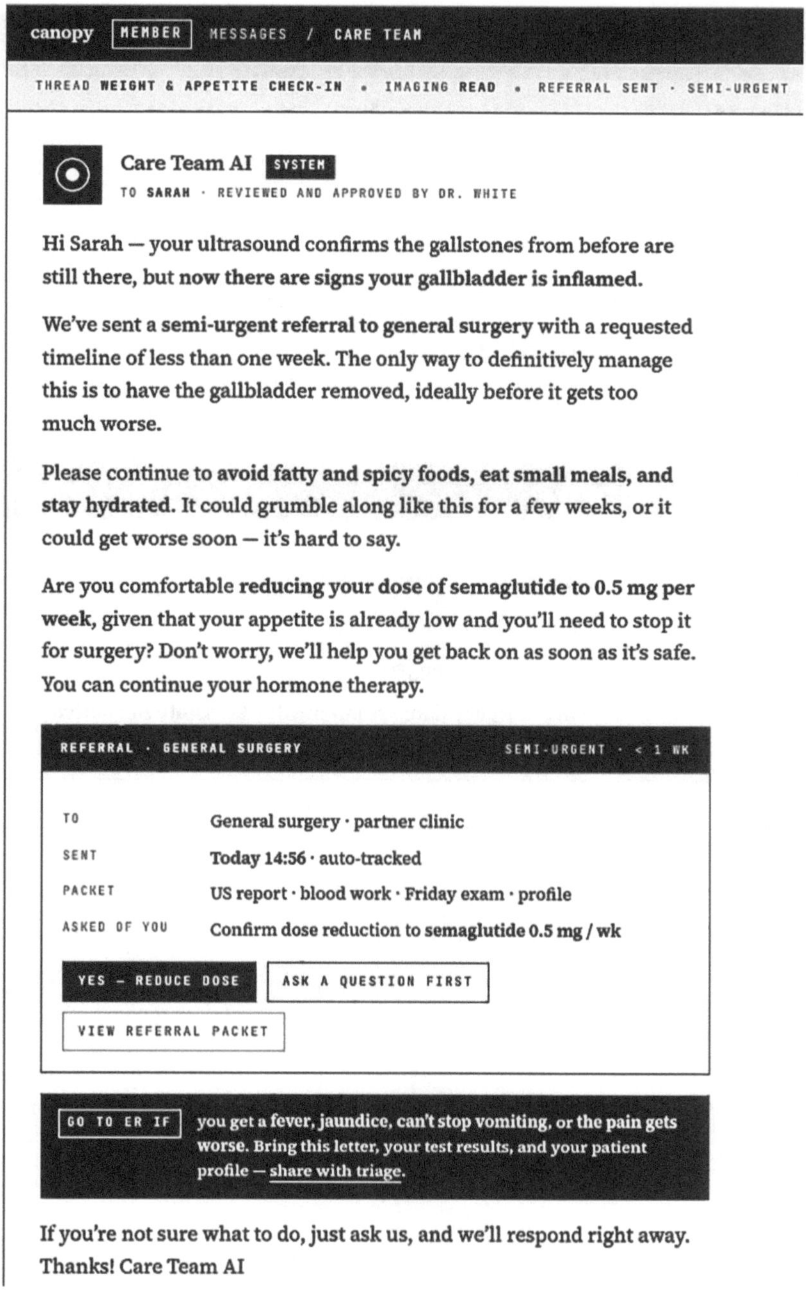

Figure 16.11 Care Team AI shares the results with Sarah.

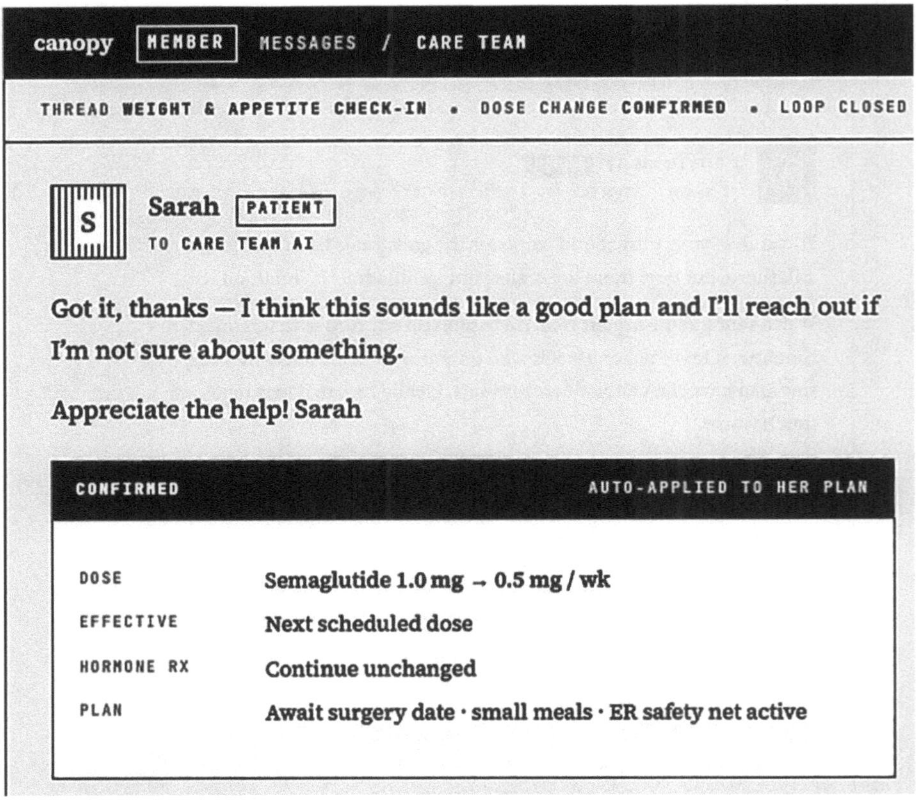

Figure 16.12 Sarah closes the loop.

PROFILE: RXFOOD—PATIENT-CENTERED NUTRITION SUPPORT

Company: RxFood
Founded: 2017
Country: Canada
Founded by: Elizabeth Choi (cofounder and CEO) and Jeff Alfonsi, MD, FRCPC, Dip ABOM, Dip ABLM (Internal Medicine/Obesity & Lifestyle Medicine)

RxFood in My Practice

Since 2023, I have used RxFood with every patient. What follows is an examination of how RxFood addresses specific gaps in obesity care delivery, particularly for patients on GLP-1 medications, and helps my patients and me make personalized decisions about their treatment.

The Right Data for Real Life

Sarah knows more about nutrition than most people. She has tried every diet framework. She used to track her intake feverishly, then stop for long stretches. The knowledge alone did not become metabolized into wisdom because it was not part of a Canopy. This is the problem with most nutrition-tracking programs: they do not integrate with other important parts of the transformation infrastructure.

What she does now is different. She logs her meals on RxFood two full days each week. If she logs her meals more than two days, she over-interprets. She has configured her view to suit this. The logging itself is fast. Most meal logs are simply a photograph from her phone. When she is moving between meetings, she sends a quick text to the platform with a few words, such as, "1 pc toast with butter and scrambled eggs made with milk" or "bowl of leftover tofu noodle stir fry," and the system captures it. For me, this is the easiest way of seeing where my patients' appetites actually are between visits.

The Q&A session Sarah attended with her cohort's dietitian in Chapter 15 is a great synchronous complement to RxFood. Sarah had been struggling for weeks to find meal inspiration that worked with her changing palate. The dietitian opened Sarah's recent RxFood log during the session, reviewed what she had actually been eating, and configured the platform to send recipes to her that fit her actual preferences and calcium goal. Sarah did not have to explain herself or remember to share screenshots. The data was already there. The recipes were already useful by the time she got home to cook.

What RxFood Does

RxFood turns meals into clinical data. Patients can photograph their food rather than manually logging it. The platform interprets those images and translates them into information a clinical team can act on: diet quality scores, nutrient balance, and intake patterns over time. RxFood makes it easy to track food and to start understanding what matters in nutrition. Patients receive personalized feedback, not generic meal plans, but specific guidance based on what they are actually eating and how it is affecting their goals. The platform can also provide recipes, food suggestions, and education tailored to each patient's needs.

The platform operates independently of electronic medical records, so programs can deploy it without waiting for IT integration. Enterprise implementation takes one week from decision to launch. Clinician training requires a single thirty-minute session.

For someone on weight-loss medication, this means answers to the questions they are asking themselves, such as which foods reduce nausea. How do you eat for satiety when appetite has collapsed? What nutrient risks emerge when appetite is over-suppressed? How do you read emotions, thoughts, and sensations as expressions of appetite?

For clinicians, RxFood removes blind spots between visits. Instead of discovering at the follow-up that a patient has been suffering, we see it in week two. We can intervene before side effects drive discontinuation.

How RxFood Helps in Early Treatment

Onboarding (Weeks 1–4)

Appetite changes immediately. Patients who previously ate three full meals suddenly feel full after four bites. Without guidance, they either force themselves to eat (and feel sick) or eat too little (and feel sick). RxFood helps patients recalibrate portion sizes, identify high-satiety foods, and understand what it means to *eat enough* when hunger signals have disappeared.

Titration (Weeks 5–12)

As doses increase, side effects intensify. Nausea, constipation, and food aversions peak during this window. This is when patients commonly abandon treatment. RxFood identifies which foods trigger nausea for each individual patient and suggests practical swaps. Not useless advice such as eat bland foods, but specific guidance based on what the patient actually tolerates and which foods have been triggering symptoms.

Side-Effect Management (Months 4–6)

Patients develop strategies tailored to their bodies. They learn which food order reduces nausea, that the timing of their fiber intake affects constipation, and that certain foods they thought were *healthy* actually make them feel worse while on medication. RxFood accelerates this learning from six months of trial and error to six weeks of guided experimentation.

Long-Term Maintenance (Months 7+)

The goal shifts from managing side effects to building sustainable habits. Patients need to maintain adequate nutrition despite reduced intake, and RxFood monitors for nutritional deficiencies that can develop over time. They need to recognize when hunger returns and what that means. They need skills that persist if they ever stop the medication. The platform transitions from intensive support to ongoing monitoring, catching problems before they become crises.

The Unit Economics

At scale, RxFood costs approximately $10 per patient per month, with unit costs declining as volume increases. Consider what it offsets:

- Clinician time spent guessing about nutrition
- Unnecessary follow-up visits for side-effect management
- Patient abandonment due to nutrition confusion
- Dietitian wait times creating treatment delays

The platform enables a digital-first, stepped-care model: immediate value, reduced barriers to access.

Empowerment, Not Compliance

RxFood builds that confidence systematically. In month one, patients gain awareness of their actual diet quality, often discovering that what they thought they were eating differs significantly from reality. By months two and three, they have learned *side-effect-awareness* eating—that is, which foods help, which hurt, and why. By months four through six, they are making autonomous meal decisions without needing constant guidance.

A few weeks after the cohort Q&A, Sarah's RxFood log starts to look different. The first set of photographs follows the dietitian's recipes, plated as written: a tofu noodle bowl on Tuesday, salmon with white beans on Thursday, and a calcium-rich yogurt parfait breakfast on the weekend. Within a month, the recipes start to drift.

She swaps the salmon for the chicken thighs she had been avoiding, because her palate is broadening again. She doubles the greens in the noodle bowl because she now likes the texture. She invents a Sunday breakfast plate she has never made before, photographs it, and the nutrient summary tells her she has built it well. Sarah is no longer following a meal plan. She is learning to nourish herself with a system that gently checks her work. It all happens on Sarah's timeline. This is what empowerment looks like when enabled by transformation infrastructure.

"We need to eat, so let's make it enjoyable and sustainable while meeting your overall goals. That is what RxFood is about."
—Dr. Jeff Alfonsi, cofounder, RxFood

ENDNOTES

1. Novo Nordisk, *State of Weight and Health Report: Unveiling Complexities of Weight, Health, Lifestyle, and Culture in America—2026 Inaugural Report*, US25OB00670 (Novo Nordisk Inc., 2026).
2. Mitchell M. Levy et al., "Surviving Sepsis Campaign: Association between Performance Metrics and Outcomes in a 7.5-Year Study," *Intensive Care Medicine* 40, no. 11 (2014): 1623–33, https://doi.org/10.1007/s00134-014-3496-0; Andrew Rhodes et al., "The Surviving Sepsis Campaign Bundles and Outcome: Results from the International Multicentre Prevalence Study on Sepsis (the IMPreSS Study)," *Intensive Care Medicine* 41, no. 9 (2015): 1620–28, https://doi.org/10.1007/s00134-015-3906-y.
3. R. Resar et al., *Using Care Bundles to Improve Health Care Quality*, IHI Innovation Series white paper (Institute for Healthcare Improvement, 2012), https://www.ihi.org/library/white-papers/using-care-bundles-improve-health-care-quality.
4. "Healthcare Solutions: Research & Engagement Platform," Evidation, https://evidation.com/for-customers/our-platform.
5. "Lilly and Evidation Health Expand Collaboration to Analyze Data from Smartphones and Connected Sensors," Eli Lilly and Company, December 14, 2018, https://investor.lilly.com/news-releases/news-release-details/lilly-and-evidation-health-expand-collaboration-analyze-data.
6. "Evidation Shares Insights on Real-World GLP-1 Dosing Behaviors," Evidation, December 16, 2025, https://evidation.com/resources/real-world-glp-1-dosing-behaviors.
7. Standards for Privacy of Individually Identifiable Health Information (HIPAA Privacy Rule), Pub. L. No. 65 FR 82,462, 45 C.F.R. Parts 160 and 164 (2000), https://www.ecfr.gov/current/title-45/part-164; 45 CFR Part 46—Protection of Human Subjects, Pub. L. No. 82 FR 7,149, 45 C.F.R. Part 46 (2017), https://www.ecfr.gov/current/title-45/part-46.

CHAPTER 17

TRANSFORMATION IN THE CANOPY

"I'm good. Really good," Sarah says.

Sarah is in my exam room for her post-operative check, four weeks after her gallbladder came out. She comes bearing no spreadsheets. No supplements in a Ziploc bag. No wearable feeds pulled up on her phone. The phone is in her bag. She doesn't need to prove to me that she is on top of it. I know she is, and the Canopy holds the data and shared truth of her case for us.

Three years ago, she worried: "*What if I can't do this on my own? What if I'm broken? What if this is just always going to be how hard it is for me to stay healthy?*"

She is not that patient anymore. She does not ask me what to do. She tells me what she is doing, what she has noticed, where she is struggling, and that she is ready to restart semaglutide after her surgery. She has updated her patient agenda and offers her thoughts on the Care plan. She wants to keep moving.

This final chapter is about what I could see was true by the end of Sarah's visit, and how I knew it. The system had done its work. It helped Sarah reach the stage of transformation where she confidently interprets her own experience, uses her resources, and asks for help more easily. That is empowerment. It is visible in her behavior, how she moves through the program, and in her clinical outcomes.

THE CANOPY, REVISITED

Empowerment occurs when the Canopy is revealed as being far greater than the sum of its components. Transformation happens over time when the components function together to create an ecosystem, and it cannot be attributed to any single one of them. The components are held in system by a mycorrhizal layer, the connective tissue of the Canopy. This allows signals to flow between components with transparency. Without it, seven components running in parallel are an expensive monocrop arranged in seven rows. With it, they function as one organism.

There are 18 system-level key performance indicators (KPIs) to measure transformation. Four are for measuring patient behavior, four for program stewardship, and 10 are validated measures of patient-centered outcomes. The KPIs are not a hierarchy or a checklist; they are a way of looking forward and looking back. A program with a Friday chart-review ritual and a spreadsheet can perform as well as a sophisticated platform with automated event routing and a data warehouse. The framework measures whether the system is producing transformation, not how it is doing so.

The Canopy framework was built for digital obesity medicine. That is where I practice, where the data are most legible, and where the architectural failures of the current market are most costly to patient health and commercial returns.

The Canopy framework generalizes easily to any other chronic disease infrastructure. Diabetes, hypertension, cardiovascular disease, mental health, and addiction all exist between doctor visits. They require the patient to manage themselves over decades inside a system designed for acute illness.

The Canopy framework generalizes further to any system designed to help humans grow and change by using programs that support adults through extended developmental arcs, programs that involve education and retraining, and programs that support recovery. The underlying challenge is the same: how do you measure whether the thing you built is creating change in the people who move through it? The KPIs contribute to that work and are reconfigurable by anyone serious about moving beyond healthcare transactions to healing transformation.

WHOLE CANOPY PATIENT BEHAVIOR KPIS

The first four whole Canopy KPIs detect the observable signs that the patient has moved through the experience and engagement tiers and toward the empowerment tier.

PAM Progression

The Patient Activation Measure® (PAM), first mentioned in Chapter 13 (see also Figure 13.1 and KPI 33), is a patient survey that "assesses an individual's knowledge, skills, and confidence integral to managing one's own health and healthcare."[1] It can be licensed from Phreesia™ for use in research, health systems, hospitals, and practices. The distance between Level 1 and Level 4 is the clinical arc that this book has been describing. We met Sarah at Level 2. We leave her at Level 4. We met Wayne at Level 1 and left him at Level 3.

KPI 33 OF 50

COMPONENT	LENS	TIER
SYSTEM	**PATIENT BEHAVIOR**	**EMPOWERMENT**

KPI **PAM® PROGRESSION**

The percentage of patients with a one-level or greater gain in Patient Activation Measure® between baseline and month 12, and the percentage of patients with PAM Level 4 attainment by month 12.

MEASURES	Whether the program produced clinically meaningful activation change in the cohort.
SIGNAL	A rising rate is indicative of activation.
TIMEFRAME	Month 12 cohort, reported monthly.

Component Breadth

The second behavioral signature is what happens to the patient's relationship with the components themselves. By incorporating more components over time, each patient configures their Canopy in a way that works for them (see KPI 34). Each additional component reduces the probability of discontinuation by more than the previous component. Subscription businesses outside healthcare have demonstrated the same pattern. Customers who engage with multiple parts of a platform have a longer, more profitable lifetime than customers who concentrate on a single product—and the effect strengthens with each additional engagement because switching costs rise with each component the customer has integrated into her routine.[2]

The trajectory matters more than the value at any single point in time. A patient whose breadth widens across the year is configuring their experience of the Canopy. If patients move from one or two components toward four or five, it signals transformation.

KPI 34 OF 50

COMPONENT	LENS	TIER
SYSTEM	**PATIENT BEHAVIOR**	**EMPOWERMENT**

KPI **COMPONENT BREADTH**

The average number of components that each active patient meaningfully engages with during a calendar month, tracked monthly across the 12-month arc.

MEASURES	Cohort-level breadth of Canopy engagement. Meaningful engagement per Component uses KPIs from those Components.
SIGNAL	A rising trajectory indicates transformation is underway.
TIMEFRAME	Monthly trajectory, with month 12 as the primary checkpoint.

Autonomy Index

The Autonomy Index instead looks for three positive indicators, all of which must be present simultaneously and sustained across months 10 through 12. The first indicator is a patient-selected self-monitoring channel maintained consistently. Sarah has several: her smart ring, her monthly weigh-in, her food log two days a week, and her journal. She chose all of them. She maintained all of them. No one is checking that she does. Wayne and Linda keep a weekly weight-and-vitals check on Friday mornings before he starts his work week, a ritual they built together. He chose it. Linda supports it. It persists.

The second indicator is at least one documented patient-initiated treatment-direction decision across the year. Sarah decided to stay at semaglutide 1 mg rather than escalate, asked for a workup for perimenopause and sleep changes, and made sure her goals of weight stability and strength were front and center. Wayne made several treatment decisions as well: the slow-titration negotiation with the Care team, receiving Linda's support, and intentionally integrating his cardiology assessment into his record.

The third indicator is component breadth of five or more.

One clarification on what *autonomy* means here. The Canopy framework does not measure whether the patient has become their own doctor. It is measuring whether the patient is doing some of the driving in her own life, which is a different thing. Autonomy in this sense draws on self-determination theory, which identifies autonomy as one of three basic psychological needs humans require for sustained motivation and well-being, alongside competence and relatedness.[3] When the need for autonomy is met, patients have better chronic disease outcomes, even within systems that do substantial clinical work on their behalf. When it is unmet, they do worse, even with excellent technical care. The Autonomy Index measures whether that need is being met (see KPI 35). Sarah is not running her care; she is participating in it. Wayne is not unsupervised; he is inside a system that has made room for his judgment.

KPI 35 OF 50

COMPONENT	LENS	TIER
SYSTEM	**PATIENT BEHAVIOR**	**EMPOWERMENT**

KPI **AUTONOMY INDEX**

The percentage of patients at month 12 who simultaneously meet three conditions, maintained across months 10 through 12.

CONDITIONS

(1) At least one patient-chosen self-monitoring channel maintained with consistency.

(2) At least one documented patient-initiated treatment-direction decision.

(3) Component breadth of 5 or more of 7.

MEASURES	Patient autonomy.
SIGNAL	Use transformation infrastructure to configure own health transformation.
TIMEFRAME	Month 12, reported monthly.

Organic Referral Rate

Wayne is at his desk when his buddy Steve calls. Steve has a question about something his doctor said near the end of his last appointment about his weight. Steve's weight has climbed over the years, and his knee pain is becoming a problem at work. That is what the appointment was about. "The doc mentioned some medication, but I honestly did not understand the rest. I know you are on something. What do you think about it?"

"The medication slows the stomach down and helps my brain catch up to my stomach," he tells Steve. "Which means you feel full a lot sooner. The first few months were hard on me, but I was just winging it. I am in a program now, and Linda is helping me stay organized, and it is going great."

Wayne goes on to say the medication is the same kind of thing as a blood pressure pill: you do not stop it when the numbers get better, because the numbers stayed better because of the medication. Steve asks for the name of the program. Wayne texts him the share link from his program profile.

That same morning, my clinic director showed me an email from Sarah. She had dinner with a colleague the previous week. The colleague mentioned that she was exhausted all the time, and her doctor kept adjusting her thyroid medication, but nothing was helping, and she did not know where else to look. She had tried to lose weight for years and was tired of trying. Sarah described the last two years of her life. The colleague asked follow-up questions. Sarah emailed the clinic director on the way home from dinner, asking if we were accepting new patients.

A rising organic referral rate signals shame reduced to a level sufficient to share, and identity changed enough to advocate (see KPI 36). Sarah's fear (revealed in Chapter 1) is gone, and she wants that for others in her life. She knows that her colleague needs to hear from someone who has done that work.

KPI 36 OF 50

COMPONENT	LENS	TIER
SYSTEM	**PATIENT BEHAVIOR**	**EMPOWERMENT**

KPI **ORGANIC REFERRAL RATE**

The share of new enrollments in a given month attributable to referrals from existing patients with no incentive, credit, or reward attached.

MEASURES	Unprompted referral as a signature of ongoing transformation.
SIGNAL	A rising rate indicates that patients have overcome enough shame to share.
TIMEFRAME	Monthly, with a rolling 12-month trailing rate.

WHOLE CANOPY PROGRAM STEWARDSHIP KPIS

The next four system-level KPIs assess whether the program is designed for the transformation measured by the whole Canopy patient behavior KPIs. Each of these KPIs is technology-agnostic by construction. The framework generalizes across diseases and across program builders. But within any disease or any builder type, the framework rewards good design over technological scale.

Individual Deviation Alert Rate

Walter Shewhart developed individual control charts in the 1920s for industrial quality control.[4] The same logic works for individual patient monitoring across hypertension, asthma, diabetes, and kidney function, with good sensitivity and specificity from a small number of data points.[5] The clinically meaningful signal is not whether a patient is above or below a population reference but whether they have deviated from their own baseline.

Sarah's gallbladder is a clear example. The signal was not that her caloric intake was low by some generic standard. The signal was low relative to her own prior baseline, and that it lasted long enough that the pattern was unlikely to be noise. The system saw it. I acted on it. She had surgery planned within a week instead of presenting to the emergency department six weeks later with a perforated gallbladder.

A small practice can produce a non-zero individual deviation alert rate for one or two variables with a well-designed chart review and a clear protocol for what counts as deviation (see KPI 37). The platform that automates this does it more efficiently and can monitor more variables. What neither can skip is the decision to look at each patient relative to themselves rather than only to the cohort. The framework rewards the design, not the tooling.

KPI 37 OF 50

COMPONENT	LENS	TIER
SYSTEM	**PROGRAM STEWARDSHIP**	**EMPOWERMENT**

KPI **INDIVIDUAL DEVIATION ALERT RATE**

The percentage of active patients in the month who had at least one alert triggered by deviation from the patient's own prior pattern.

MEASURES	Whether the program detects change against each patient's own established pattern. Technology-agnostic.
SIGNAL	A program with personal-baseline detection will report a sustained non-zero rate.
TIMEFRAME	Monthly.

Program Step Change Rate

A program must calibrate intensity to where a patient actually is, so as not to overshoot when they do not need support, nor undershoot when they do. Service intensity moves in both directions, and a functioning program shows both directions in the data every month. A step-up is more intensive for a component than the prior month: an increase in coaching frequency, an additional clinical visit, or a new Curriculum module sequenced into the patient's plan (see KPI 38). A step-down is less intensive: a coaching cadence reduction as a patient stabilizes, a transition from active to maintenance Care, or a move from weekly to monthly weight and vital sign checks.

Component Cross-Reference Rate

Sarah's gallbladder journey referenced three Components in a single week. Connection detected the pattern in her food log and her wearable data. Care received the alert, drew my attention, ordered the workup, and managed the surgical referral. Curriculum delivered the post-operative nutrition module before her surgery date. One event in one component triggered an action in two others. That is integration (see KPI 39). It is also what kept her out of the emergency department.

Cohort-Over-Cohort Improvement Rate

The last whole Canopy program-stewardship KPI compares the current enrollment cohort to the cohort enrolled six months earlier (see KPI 40). If the current cohort is outperforming the prior cohort on a meaningful share of patient-behavior KPIs, the program is learning and improving alongside the patients. If the current cohort is performing the same or worse, the program has not embedded learning and the metrics it reports each month are static descriptions of a static program. The comparison needs to be controlled for baseline characteristics to avoid rewarding selection of *easier* patients.

This KPI measures whether, in the six months before any new patient arrives, the program changed something that made the experience better for patients like them. It shows whether the program is doing the work of getting better.

KPI 38 OF 50

COMPONENT	LENS	TIER
SYSTEM	**PROGRAM STEWARDSHIP**	**EMPOWERMENT**

KPI **PROGRAM STEP CHANGE RATE**

The percentage of active patients in the month whose documented service intensity changed (up or down) versus the prior month, across five Components (Care, Curriculum, Coach, Community, Connection). Cost and Coverage excluded.

MEASURES	Whether the program is calibrating service intensity to patient need. The total rate is reported with step-ups and step-downs broken out separately.
SIGNAL	Both step-ups and step-downs are visible every month in the cohort.
TIMEFRAME	Monthly. One transition up and/or down counted per patient per Component per month.

KPI 39 OF 50

COMPONENT	LENS	TIER
SYSTEM	**PROGRAM STEWARDSHIP**	**EMPOWERMENT**

KPI **COMPONENT CROSS-REFERENCE RATE**

The percentage of active patients in the month for whom at least one action in one Component was triggered by data or an event originating in another Component.

MEASURES	Designed integration across the Components.
SIGNAL	A program with siloed Components is not leveraging the Canopy.
TIMEFRAME	Monthly. One cross-Component trigger counted per patient per month.

KPI 40 OF 50

COMPONENT	LENS	TIER
SYSTEM	**PROGRAM STEWARDSHIP**	**EMPOWERMENT**

KPI **COHORT-OVER-COHORT IMPROVEMENT RATE**

The share of the program's published patient behavior KPIs (Component-level and system-level) where the current enrollment cohort is outperforming the cohort enrolled six months earlier, measured at the same post-enrollment tenure, and controlling for baseline characteristics.

MEASURES	Whether program learning is producing measurable cohort-level gains. Aggregated across all cohort members, not a curated subset.
SIGNAL	Sustained rises indicate learning is embedded into the program.
TIMEFRAME	Monthly. Comparison cohort enrolled six months prior, each measured at current tenure.

WHAT ABOUT WEIGHT?

You may be wondering why I have not spent more of this book emphasizing how much weight patients should lose. The reasons are myriad, but the one that matters most is this: we can lose weight without becoming healthier or our lives getting any better. If that weight loss is not connected to an experience of transformation, no matter how small, it will not endure. It does not matter how effective the medications are or how cheap they get. Weight is an insufficient marker of progress here.

The 10 KPIs that follow are anchored to the International Consortium for Health Outcomes Measurement (ICHOM) adult obesity standard set, the international consensus on what outcomes matter to patients and clinicians in adult obesity care.[6] The ICHOM panel includes clinicians and patients across more than twenty countries. Where validated instruments exist, the framework uses them. Where ICHOM has acknowledged a measurement gap, the framework names the closest available proxy. I chose 10 outcomes based on how easy they are to capture across multiple practice settings without large capital investments in diagnostic equipment or the requirement for laboratory testing.

BMI Change and Waist-to-Height Ratio

Body mass index (BMI) is in the ICHOM dataset, but I have modified it here to BMI change (see KPI 41). It captures what most patients and most payers look at first. Sarah achieved a 14% total weight loss from her highest adult weight and maintained it through her surgical recovery and beyond. Wayne lost over 15% of his total weight and has maintained it. These losses are significant to Sarah and Wayne and meet the threshold of clinical significance.

Waist-to-height ratio (WHtR) (see KPI 42) adds a measure of specificity to BMI by estimating visceral fat. Visceral adiposity (fat), not total body weight, is the primary driver of cardiovascular and metabolic risk. A tape measure at the umbilicus, divided by height, is patient-reportable and costs almost nothing. It is also one of the outcomes most predictive of cardiometabolic improvement independent of BMI.[7]

KPI 41 OF 50

COMPONENT	LENS	TIER
SYSTEM	**OUTCOME**	**EMPOWERMENT**

KPI **BMI CHANGE**

The change in body mass index (BMI, kg/m^2) from baseline, reported as percent change in body weight and as absolute change.

MEASURES	The composite body-composition response to treatment.
TIMEFRAME	Baseline, then monthly, with annual as the outcome checkpoint for the KPI.

KPI 42 OF 50

COMPONENT	LENS	TIER
SYSTEM	**OUTCOME**	**EMPOWERMENT**

KPI **WAIST-TO-HEIGHT RATIO**

The change in the ratio of waist circumference to height from baseline, with both measurements in the same units.

MEASURES	Visceral adiposity reduction, the metabolic-risk fraction of weight loss. Patient-reportable; no specialized equipment required.
TIMEFRAME	Baseline and monthly, with annual as the outcome checkpoint.

General Quality of Life

Sarah's mobility, pain, and anxiety dimensions all improved over the measurement period (see KPI 43). She can cross her legs comfortably now. She sleeps through the night with her hormone therapy in place. During a recent visit, she described herself as less afraid of the future. Wayne's mobility and self-care dimensions improved as his weight stabilized and his joint function returned. Getting in and out of his car is not as much of an effort as it was two years ago.

The EQ-5D-5L is a five-dimension patient-reported outcome measure that captures mobility, self-care, usual activities, pain and discomfort, and anxiety and depression.[8]

Sleep Apnea

The STOP-Bang questionnaire is a brief, eight-item clinical screening tool that estimates a patient's risk of obstructive sleep apnea using snoring, tiredness, observed apnea, blood pressure, BMI, age, neck circumference, and sex.[9] Untreated obstructive sleep apnea dysregulates appetite hormones, raises insulin resistance, and elevates cardiovascular and metabolic risk, and the resulting sleep fragmentation makes weight loss measurably harder to achieve[10] (see KPI 44).

Eating Behavior and Body Image

Eating behavior (see KPI 45) is a patient-reported outcome that captures how a patient relates to food, hunger, and satiety. Changes in eating behavior predict whether weight loss can be sustained. Patient-reported tools that capture how a patient eats, rather than only what they eat, are rare.

The BODY-Q eating behavior scale is a subset scale of the larger BODY-Q instrument and is one of the few that produces clinically actionable information.[11] The BODY-Q eating behavior scale measures appetite regulation, control over portions, satisfaction after eating, grazing between meals, eating pace, and the quality of food choices. The full BODY-Q library contains 31 independently functioning scales. Six of the scales were selected by expert consensus for use in the ICHOM adult obesity standard set.[12]

KPI 43 OF 50

COMPONENT	LENS	TIER
SYSTEM	**OUTCOME**	**EMPOWERMENT**

KPI **GENERAL QUALITY OF LIFE**

The change in the EQ-5D-5L composite index score from baseline, with each of the five dimensions reported as a diagnostic breakdown.

MEASURES	Patient self-reported quality of life across the five dimensions. Instrument: EQ-5D-5L.
TIMEFRAME	Baseline, six months, and month 12, then annually.

KPI 44 OF 50

COMPONENT	LENS	TIER
SYSTEM	**OUTCOME**	**EMPOWERMENT**

KPI **SLEEP APNEA**

The change in STOP-Bang screening score from baseline, including movement across risk strata (low, intermediate, high).

MEASURES	Obstructive sleep apnea risk and sleep quality as a downstream signal of metabolic, cardiovascular, and mental-health improvement. Instrument: STOP-Bang.
TIMEFRAME	Baseline, six months, and month 12, then annually.

KPI 45 OF 50

COMPONENT	LENS	TIER
SYSTEM	**OUTCOME**	**EMPOWERMENT**

KPI **EATING BEHAVIOR**

The change in BODY-Q Eating Behavior Scale score from baseline.

MEASURES	**The patient's self-reported relationship with eating, including appetite regulation, satiety, portion control, grazing, eating pace, and food quality. Instrument: BODY-Q Obesity Module, Eating Behavior Scale.**
TIMEFRAME	**Baseline, six months, and month 12, then annually.**

A Note on Big Eating

In my practice, I do not use terms such as *control*, *restraint*, or *emotional eating* with patients. These words carry decades of diet-culture baggage, and what they actually describe is eating that happens outside of planned structure, or eating that responds to internal states or genetics. Neither is about control or worth.

I use *big eating* instead because it is practical and neutral. It allows a level-set conversation without importing judgment. A patient who hears *uncontrolled eating* hears a verdict on their character, which does not belong in the therapeutic relationship. A patient who hears *big eating* hears a description of what happened.

Many instruments used to measure eating behavior use these terms as they are clinical language. This may be appropriate for psychometric purposes, but they do not need to be used in patient-facing language.

Body image (see KPI 46) is a patient-reported outcome that captures how a patient feels about their body. Body image dissatisfaction predicts disordered eating, treatment dropout, and weight regain. Improvements in body satisfaction independently track with sustained weight loss, which means body image is not a cosmetic outcome.[13]

The BODY-Q body image scale measures satisfaction with body shape and size, comfort with how the body looks clothed and unclothed, and the degree of worry or anxiety the patient experiences about their appearance.

COMPONENT	LENS	TIER
SYSTEM	**OUTCOME**	**EMPOWERMENT**

KPI **BODY IMAGE**

The change in BODY-Q Body Image Scale score from baseline.

MEASURES	The patient's self-reported satisfaction with body shape, size, and appearance, and the degree of worry or anxiety associated with how their body looks. Instrument: BODY-Q Obesity Module, Body Image Scale.
TIMEFRAME	Baseline, six months, and month 12, then annually.

Mental Health

Depression (see KPI 47) and obesity have a bidirectional relationship: depression increases the risk of obesity through reduced activity, disrupted sleep, dysregulated appetite, and weight-gain side effects of antidepressant medications. Obesity increases the risk of depression through systemic inflammation, weight stigma, and reduced quality of life. Treating one without screening for the other risks missing their connection.

The PHQ-9 is a nine-item patient-reported instrument that screens for the severity of depression symptoms by asking how often the patient has experienced each symptom over the prior two weeks.[14]

Anxiety (see KPI 48) dysregulates appetite and stress hormones and is associated with disordered eating patterns. Untreated anxiety predicts patient dropout from weight loss programs and from medication treatment, which makes it a screening priority for any program managing chronic disease over time.[15] The GAD-7 is a seven-item patient-reported instrument that screens for the severity of symptoms present in generalized anxiety disorder. It asks about core anxiety symptoms over the prior two weeks, including excessive worry, restlessness, difficulty relaxing, and irritability.

KPI 47 OF 50

COMPONENT	LENS	TIER
SYSTEM	**OUTCOME**	**EMPOWERMENT**

KPI **DEPRESSION**

The change in PHQ-9 score from baseline, including movement across severity strata (none, mild, moderate, moderately severe, severe).

MEASURES	Depression severity as a downstream mental-health signal. Instrument: Patient Health Questionnaire 9-item (PHQ-9).
TIMEFRAME	Baseline, six months, and month 12, then annually.

COMPONENT	LENS	TIER
SYSTEM	**OUTCOME**	**EMPOWERMENT**

KPI **ANXIETY**

The change in GAD-7 score from baseline, including movement across severity strata (minimal, mild, moderate, severe).

MEASURES	Generalized anxiety severity as a downstream mental-health signal. Instrument: Generalized Anxiety Disorder 7-item (GAD-7).
TIMEFRAME	Baseline, six months, and month 12, then annually.

Internalized Weight Bias

Think of internalized weight bias as part of the pathology of obesity. In 2024, a 72-week behavioral weight-loss trial of 105 adults with high internalized weight bias revealed that the participants whose internalized bias scores decreased during the first 20 weeks lost significantly more weight at week 46 than participants whose scores remained elevated. This was independent of physical activity.[16]

Any form of bias, stigma, or discrimination is a stressor that affects how people heal and receive help. Internalized weight bias is independently associated with disordered eating, depression, anxiety, exercise avoidance, treatment dropout, and worse weight-loss outcomes, even after controlling for BMI and for experienced stigma.[17] It is a clinically meaningful target in its own right and not a downstream consequence of body size. In fact, it is more likely that body size is downstream of internalized weight bias. This means that it may still be there when the weight comes down.

By this point in the book, it should be clear that language is a clinical intervention, of sorts. The way a program frames the disease of obesity gets internalized by patients over months of exposure to the words it uses to describe eating, the way it talks about weight regain, the mention of possible side effects, and the patient's role in their own care.

The Weight Bias Internalization Scale (WBIS) is an 11-item patient-reported scale that measures the extent to which a patient applies negative weight-related stereotypes to themselves (see KPI 49). It is self-directed weight bias rather than bias from external sources or experiences.[18] The ICHOM acknowledges a gap in this area in terms of how to measure it, so I recommend the WBIS to evaluate and track internalized weight bias. Reductions on the WBIS do not happen by accident. There is no shortcut to this outcome. It is the dividend of having taken the language of obesity medicine seriously from day one.

KPI **49** OF 50

COMPONENT	LENS	TIER
SYSTEM	**OUTCOME**	**EMPOWERMENT**

KPI **INTERNALIZED WEIGHT BIAS**

The change in the Weight Bias Internalization Scale (WBIS) score from baseline.

MEASURES	Patient self-directed weight stigma. Instrument: WBIS, an 11-item validated patient-reported instrument used as the closest available proxy for the ICHOM-acknowledged measurement gap.
TIMEFRAME	Baseline, six months, and month 12, then annually.

Adverse Event Rate—Due to Program Interventions

Adverse events are part of every effective treatment, and obesity medications are no exception. It is a matter of when, not if. Adverse events are undesirable experiences associated with obesity treatment where the patient outcome is one of six things: death, life-threatening illness, hospitalization, disability or permanent damage, a need for ongoing medical attention, or another serious medical event. Adverse events should be continuously captured, and any component can receive the adverse event signal. Programs can define additional adverse events that reflect broader threats to patient success.

The ICHOM Adult Obesity Standard Set specifies the variables that should be captured, and they are narrowly focused on medication-related adverse events: all-cause mortality, vascular complications, self-harm or suicidal ideations, dumping syndrome, internal hemorrhage, pulmonary or cardiac problems, malnutrition, ulcer, gallstones, bowel obstruction, hypoglycemia, pancreatitis, thyroid cancer, and others.[19] These match quite closely with adverse event reporting requirements for drug regulators. However, treatment is not the same as medication. Additional variables can be defined for other interventions at the program level.

This KPI is where program stewardship KPIs (mentioned earlier in this chapter) do their regulatory work. The individual deviation alert rate can detect an impending event relative to a patient's baseline (see KPI 50). The component cross-reference rate routes the signal from Connection to Care to Curriculum so the response is coordinated rather than fragmented. The program step change rate calibrates the response intensity to what the patient actually needs.

KPI 50 OF 50

COMPONENT	LENS	TIER
SYSTEM	OUTCOME	EMPOWERMENT

KPI ADVERSE EVENT RATE – PROGRAM INTERVENTIONS

The change from baseline in the per-patient rate of serious adverse events attributable to program interventions, reported as an overall rate with categorical breakdown across interventions. For the obesity medication intervention category, the ICHOM-specified adverse event type must be captured.

MEASURES	**Intervention-related harm detected by intervention category and adverse event type.**
TIMEFRAME	**Continuously captured, with cohort-level reporting every month.**

AN INVITATION TO THE CANOPY

Sarah is not broken. But our healthcare systems are. The monocrop model will not solve the problems that are before us.

Historically, resistance to designing and building for patient success has been structural. The assumption was a trade-off: that the moves a clinician would make to improve the patient's life were the moves a CFO would have to overrule in the name of the business. The Canopy shows that no such trade-off exists in obesity medicine. Long-term value is long-term health. The metrics that detect transformation are the same metrics that predict commercial durability. There is no version of the data in which one metric moves while the others do not, especially over the long term. That is, as long as you are aiming for wallet share.

If you are leading an existing obesity medicine program, the invitation is not to completely rebuild in one quarter. It is smaller and more specific: pick two or three Canopy KPIs that match where you already are. Start with a problem you are facing that belongs in the clinical last mile, or second moment of truth. Get really specific about where you want to improve and start measuring it now. Ask your patients about their experiences and points of view. Ask them if they would be interested in participating in some of the aforementioned programs in the name of improving the quality of your offer.

Resist the temptation to pick a weight loss trend, throw a shiny little product feature at it, and further commodify your program into a collection of little add-ons. The market has enough of those. That is exactly how we got into this mess, in digital health and in medicine. This is the monocrop problem.

Instead, solve for the forest. Pick a meaningful metric and use your insights to start building real components, solid trunks to return those insights to the transformation of your patients. Once you start succeeding on a few metrics, adding more is enticing because ecosystems are self-reinforcing, requiring fewer and fewer inputs for each marginal gain.

The Canopy is open. And so is the invitation to build it together.

ENDNOTES

1. "Patient Activation Measure® (PAM®)," Insignia Health (a Phreesia™ Company), February 14, 2025, https://www.insigniahealth.com/pam/.
2. Werner J. Reinartz and V. Kumar, "The Impact of Customer Relationship Characteristics on Profitable Lifetime Duration," *Journal of Marketing* 67, no. 1 (2003): 77–99, https://doi.org/10.1509/jmkg.67.1.77.18589; Rajkumar Venkatesan and V. Kumar, "A Customer Lifetime Value Framework for Customer Selection and Resource Allocation Strategy," *Journal of Marketing* 68, no. 4 (2004): 106–25, https://doi.org/10.1509/jmkg.68.4.106.42728.
3. R. M. Ryan and E. L. Deci, "Self-Determination Theory and the Facilitation of Intrinsic Motivation, Social Development, and Well-Being," *The American Psychologist* 55, no. 1 (2000): 68–78, https://doi.org/10.1037//0003-066x.55.1.68; Johan Y. Y. Ng et al., "Self-Determination Theory Applied to Health Contexts: A Meta-Analysis," *Perspectives on Psychological Science: A Journal of the Association for Psychological Science* 7, no. 4 (2012): 325–40, https://doi.org/10.1177/1745691612447309.
4. Walter A. Stewhart, *Economic Control of Quality of Manufactured Product* (Van Nostrand, 1931).
5. Ruth Tennant et al., "Monitoring Patients Using Control Charts: A Systematic Review," *International Journal for Quality in Health Care: Journal of the International Society for Quality in Health Care* 19, no. 4 (2007): 187–94, https://doi.org/10.1093/intqhc/mzm015.
6. International Consortium for Health Outcomes Measurement, "Adult Obesity," *ICHOM*, n.d., accessed May 9, 2026, https://www.ichom.org/patient-centered-outcome-measure/adult-obesity/.
7. M. Ashwell et al., "Waist-to-Height Ratio Is a Better Screening Tool than Waist Circumference and BMI for Adult Cardiometabolic Risk Factors: Systematic Review and Meta-Analysis," *Obesity Reviews: An Official Journal of the International Association for the Study of Obesity* 13, no. 3 (2012): 275–86, https://doi.org/10.1111/j.1467-789X.2011.00952.x.
8. M. Herdman et al., "Development and Preliminary Testing of the New Five-Level Version of EQ-5D (EQ-5D-5L)," *Quality of Life Research* 20, no. 10 (2011): 1727–36, https://doi.org/10.1007/s11136-011-9903-x.
9. Frances Chung et al., "STOP Questionnaire: A Tool to Screen Patients for Obstructive Sleep Apnea," *Anesthesiology* 108, no. 5 (2008): 812–21, https://doi.org/10.1097/ALN.0b013e31816d83e4.
10. Sirimon Reutrakul and Eve Van Cauter, "Sleep Influences on Obesity, Insulin Resistance, and Risk of Type 2 Diabetes," *Metabolism—Clinical and Experimental* 84 (July 2018): 56–66, https://doi.org/10.1016/j.metabol.2018.02.010.
11. Simon W. Nienhuijs et al., "Dutch Nationwide Cohort Experience with a New PROMs Set in Metabolic and Bariatric Surgery: BODY-Q Obesity Module," *Obesity Surgery* 35 (2024): 67–77.

12. Teferi Mekonnen et al., "Development of a Core Patient-Centred Outcome Set for Adults Living with Obesity: A Modified Delphi-Based International Consensus," *eClinicalMedicine* 87 (2025): 103422.
13. Natascha-Alexandra Weinberger et al., "Body Dissatisfaction in Individuals with Obesity Compared to Normal-Weight Individuals: A Systematic Review and Meta-Analysis," *Obesity Facts* 9, no. 6 (2016): 424–41, https://doi.org/10.1159/000454837; António L. Palmeira et al., "Change in Body Image and Psychological Well-Being During Behavioral Obesity Treatment: Associations with Weight Loss and Maintenance," *Body Image* 7, no. 3 (2010): 187–93, https://doi.org/10.1016/j.bodyim.2010.03.002; I. Moroshko, L. Brennan, and P. O'Brien, "Predictors of Dropout in Weight Loss Interventions: A Systematic Review of the Literature," *Obesity Reviews* 12, no. 11 (2011): 912–34, https://doi.org/10.1111/j.1467-789X.2011.00915.x; David B. Sarwer, J. Kevin Thompson, and Thomas F. Cash, "Body Image and Obesity in Adulthood," *Psychiatric Clinics of North America* 28, no. 1 (2005): 69–87, https://doi.org/10.1016/j.psc.2004.09.002.
14. K. Kroenke et al., "The PHQ-9: Validity of a Brief Depression Severity Measure," *Journal of General Internal Medicine* 16, no. 9 (2001): 606–13, https://doi.org/10.1046/j.1525-1497.2001.016009606.x.
15. Floriana S. Luppino et al., *Overweight, Obesity, and Depression A Systematic Review and Meta-Analysis of Longitudinal Studies*, n.d., https://doi.org/67(3):220–229.
16. Miriam Sheynblyum et al., "Longitudinal Associations of Internalized Weight Stigma with Physical Activity and Weight Loss," *Obesity Science & Practice* 10, no. 4 (2024): e773, https://doi.org/10.1002/osp4.773.
17. R. L. Pearl and R. M. Puhl, "Weight Bias Internalization and Health: A Systematic Review," *Obesity Reviews* 19, no. 8 (2018): 1141–63, https://doi.org/10.1111/obr.12701.
18. Laura E. Durso and Janet D. Latner, "Understanding Self-Directed Stigma: Development of the Weight Bias Internalization Scale," *Obesity* 16, no. S2 (2008): S80–86, https://doi.org/10.1038/oby.2008.448.
19. International Consortium for Health Outcomes Measurement, "Adult Obesity."

INDEX

Note: page numbers set in italic refer to figures